THE LEAN & GREEN LOW CARB DIET COOKBOOK

AN INCLUSIVE GUIDE ON JUST HOW TO LOSE WEIGHT, LIVE HEATHY, AND RESET YOUR METABOLISM. INSIDE AN AFFORDABLE DIET PLAN THAT INCLUDES QUICK, EASY, DELICIOUS LEAN AND GREEN RECIPES.

EMMA J. LAWRENCE

Legal & Disclaimer

The information contained in this book and its contents is not designed to replace or take the place of any form of medical or professional advice; and is not meant to replace the need for independent medical, financial, legal or other professional advice or services, as may be required. The content and information in this book has been provided for educational and entertainment purposes only.

The content and information contained in this book has been compiled from sources deemed reliable, and it is accurate to the best of the Author's knowledge, information and belief. However, the Author cannot guarantee its accuracy and validity and cannot be held liable for any errors and/or omissions. Further, changes are periodically made to this book as and when needed. Where appropriate and/or necessary, you must consult a professional (including but not limited to your doctor, attorney, financial advisor or such other professional advisor) before using any of the suggested remedies, techniques, or information in this book.

4

Table of Contents

Introduction of Low Carb Lean & Green diet

Following the Low Carb program requires you to eat low-calorie, low-carb foods. If you don't like to cook or are a busy person, and don't have enough time to cook your meals, the Low Carb diet will be great for you as it doesn't require you to do any prolonged cooking and is easy to execute.

The Low Carb diet improves weight loss through meals known as "Fuelings", while homemade entrées are called "Lean and Green" meals.

Fuelings consists of meals that are specifically low in carbohydrates but high in protein.

To record success with this diet plan, you need to stick to the Fuelings, which are supplemented with vegetables, meat and healthy fats every day; you will be full and nourished. Although you will consume few calories, you won't lose a lot of muscle because you will be nourished with a lot of fiber, protein and other vital nutrients. Your calories as an adult will not exceed 800 to 1,000. You can lose 12 pounds in 12 weeks if you follow the Optimal Weight 5&1 Plan option.

Since you reduce your carbohydrate intake in this diet plan, fat will be eliminated naturally because carbohydrate is the primary source of energy, so if it is not readily available, the body finds a fat alternative, which implies that the body will have to break down fat for energy and keep burning fat.

This diet plan tilts towards being a favorite among various people with such a busy lifestyle, but the low-calorie approach of the diet plan is proposed for anyone who wants to lose that excess weight.

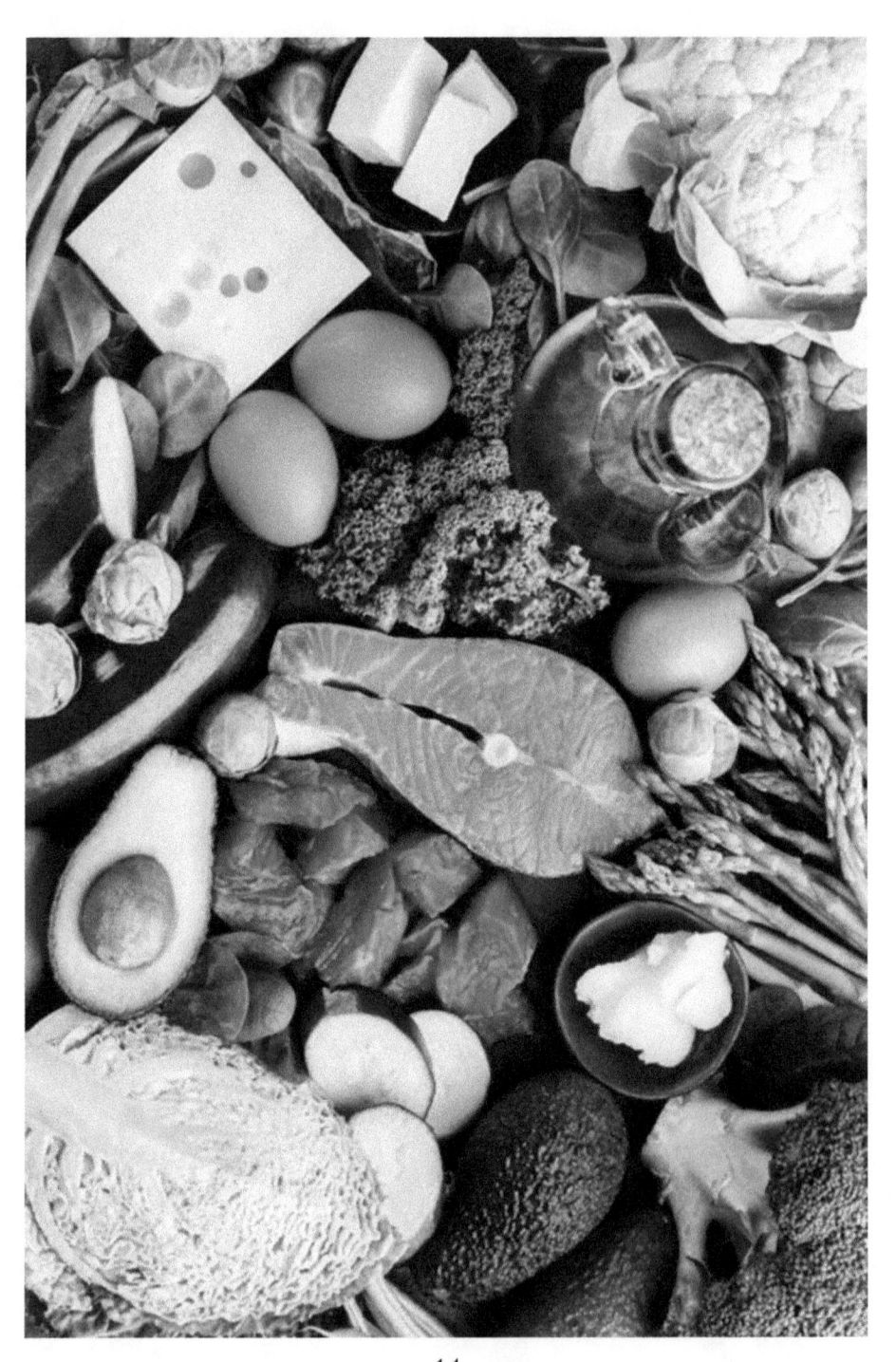

Chapter 1: What Is the Low Carb Lean & Green diet?

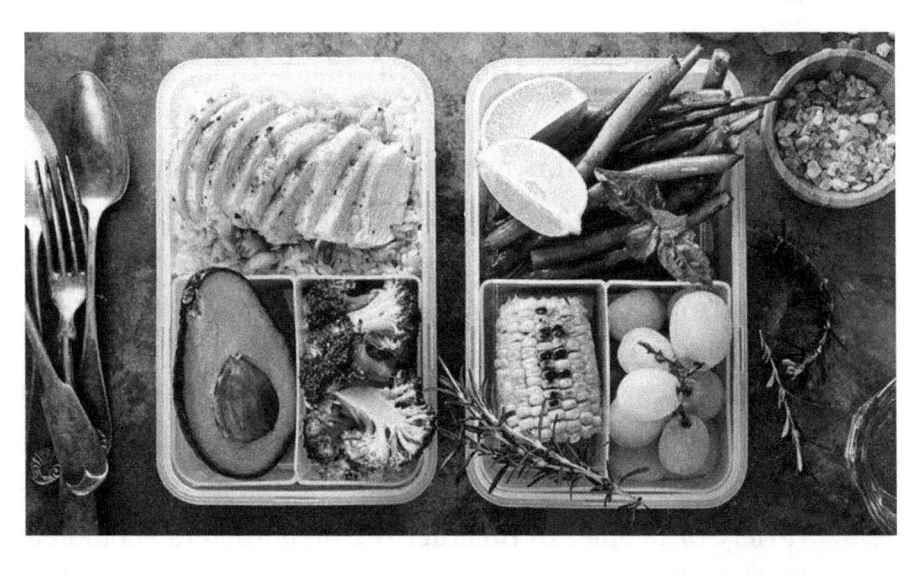

The Low Carb Lean and Green diet encourages people to limit the number of calories they should consume daily. Under this program, dieters are encouraged to consume between 800 and 1000 calories per day. For this to be possible, dieters are encouraged to opt for healthier food items and meal replacements. But unlike other types of commercial diet regimens, the Low Carb Lean and Green diet is available in several variations. There are currently three variants of the Low Carb Lean and Green Diet plan that you can choose based on your needs.

- **5&1 Low Carb Diet Plan:** This is the most common version of this diet, and it involves eating five Fuelings meals and a balanced homemade dinner Lean and Green.

- **4&2&1 Low Carb Diet Plan:** his diet plan is designed for people who want to have flexibility while following this regimen. Under this program, dieters are encouraged to eat more calories and have more flexible food choices. This means they can eat four Fueling meals, three homemade meals from Lean and Green recipes and one snack per day.

- **5&2&2 Low Carb Diet Plan:** This diet plan is perfect for individuals who prefer to have a flexible meal plan to achieve a healthy weight. It is recommended for a wide variety of people. In this diet regimen, dieters should eat five meals, two lean and green meals, and two healthy snacks.

- **3&3 Low Carb Diet Plan:** This particular diet plan is created for people who have moderate weight issues and simply want to maintain a healthy body. Under this diet plan, dieters are encouraged to eat three Fuelings meals and three Lean and Green meals.

- **Low Carb Lean and Green diet for Nursing Mothers:** This diet regimen is designed for nursing mothers with babies at least two months old. In addition to supporting nursing mothers, it also encourages progressive weight loss.

- **Low Carb Lean and Green diet for Diabetes:** This diet plan is designed for people with type 1 and 2 diabetes. The meal plans are designed for people to consume more green and lean meals depending on their needs and conditions.

- **Low Carb Lean and Green diet for Gout:** This diet regimen incorporates a balance of low in purines and moderate in protein.

- **Low Carb Lean and Green diet for seniors (65 years and older):** Designed for seniors, this Low Carb diet plan has some variations following Fuelings ingredients depending on the needs and activities of the dieting seniors.

- **Low Carb Lean and Green diet for Teen Boys and Teen Girls (13–18 years old):** Planned for active teens, Low Carb Lean and Green diet for Teens Boys and Teens Girls provide the right nutrition to growing teens.

- Regardless of which type of diet plan you choose, you must talk with a coach to identify which program is right for you based on your individual goals. This is to ensure that you get the most out of the problem you choose.

How Does the Low Carb Lean & Green Diet Work?

Most people follow the 5&1 program which incorporates 5 refills per day.

On this program, clients eat 5 Fuelings meals and 1 Lean and Green homemade low-calorie meal per day.

You can choose from more than 60 options, including smoothies, soups, and puddings. Your sixth daily meal (which you can eat anytime) is built around 3 servings of non-starchy vegetables, cooked lean protein and healthy fats.

Once you reach your weight goal, the transition off the plan should be more comfortable as your old habits are replaced with healthier ones.

For people who want a more flexible, high-calorie diet, we suggest the 4&2&1 plan, which incorporates 4 meals, 2 lean, green meals, and 1 healthy snack, such as a serving of baked potatoes or fruit.

There are also specific programs for people with diabetes, nursing moms, seniors, and teens, which will be explained in future dedicated publications.

Chapter 2: Compliant and Noncompliant Food

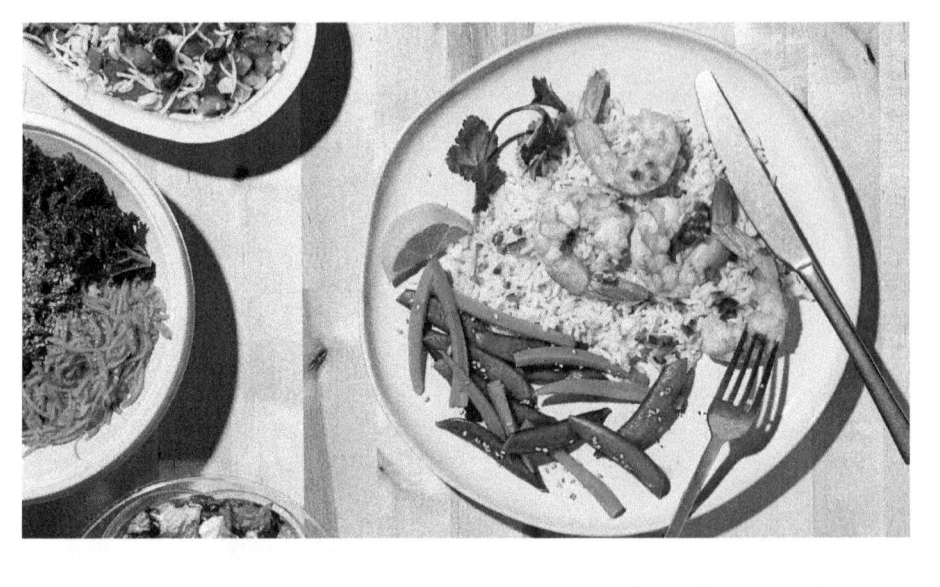

There are so many foods that you can eat while following the Low Carb Lean and Green Diet. However, you must know these foods by heart. This is especially true if you are just new to this diet, and you have to strictly follow the 5&1 Low Carb Diet Plan. Thus, this is dedicated to the types of foods you are allowed and not allowed to eat while following this diet regimen.

The majority of the food you will be consuming on the Low Carb diet's strategies comes directly from the corporation, but you will also need to buy products to make up for your Lean and Green meal of the day.

Compliant Foods

There are several categories of foods that can be eaten under this diet regimen. We will break down the Lean and Green foods that you can eat while following this diet regime.

Fuelings

You can select from over 60 soups, shakes, brownies, etc. as meal Fuelings.

The Lean Foods

Leanest Foods: These foods are considered to be the leanest as it has only up to 4 grams of total fat. Moreover, dieters should eat a 7-ounce cooked portion of these foods. Consume these foods with 1 healthy fat serving. These include the following:

- **Fish:** Flounder, cod, haddock, grouper, Mahi, tilapia, tuna (yellowfin fresh or canned), and wild catfish

- **Shellfish:** Scallops, lobster, crabs, shrimp

- **Game meat:** Elk, deer, buffalo

- **Ground turkey or other meat:** Should be 98% lean

- **Meatless alternatives:** 14 egg whites, 2 cups egg substitute, 5 ounces' seitan, 1 ½ cups 1% cottage cheese, and 12 ounces non-fat 0% Greek yogurt

Leaner Foods: These foods contain 5 to 9 grams of total fat. Consume these foods with 1 healthy fat serving. Make sure to consume only 6 ounces of a cooked portion of these foods daily.

- **Fish:** Halibut, trout, and swordfish

- **Chicken:** White meat such as breasts as long as the skin is removed

- **Turkey:** Ground turkey as long as it is 95 to 97% lean

- **Meatless options:** 2 whole eggs plus 4 egg whites, 2 whole eggs plus one cup egg substitute, 1 ½ cups 2% cottage cheese, and 12 ounces low fat 2% plain Greek yogurt

Lean Foods: These are foods that contain 10 to 20 g of total fat. When consuming these foods, there should be no serving of healthy fat. These include the following:

- **Fish:** Tuna (Bluefin steak), salmon, herring, farmed catfish, and mackerel

- **Lean beef:** Ground, steak, and roast

- **Lamb:** All cuts

- **Pork:** Pork chops, pork tenderloin, and all parts. Make sure to remove the skin

- **Ground turkey and other meats:** 85 to 94% lean

- **Chicken:** Any dark meat

- **Meatless Options:** 15 ounces extra-firm tofu, 3 whole eggs (up to two times per week), 4 ounces reduced-fat skim cheese, 8 ounces part-skim ricotta cheese, and 5 ounces tempeh

Healthy Fat Servings: Healthy fat servings are allowed under this diet. They should contain 5 grams of fat and fewer grams of carbohydrates. Regardless of what type of Low Carb Diet plan you follow, make sure that you add between 0 and 2 healthy fat servings daily. Below are the different healthy fat servings that you can eat:

- 1 teaspoon oil (any kind of oil)

- 1 tablespoon low carbohydrate salad dressing

- 2 tablespoons reduced-fat salad dressing

- 5 to 10 black or green olives

- 1 ½ ounce avocado

- 1/3 ounce plain nuts including peanuts, almonds, pistachios

- 1 tablespoon plain seeds such as chia, sesame, flax, and pumpkin seeds

- ½ tablespoon regular butter, mayonnaise, and margarine

The Green and Non-Starchy Foods

Low Carb's 5&1 plan permits for 2 non-starchy vegetables together with the protein in your Lean and Green meal.

The vegetables are allocated into lower, moderate, and higher carbohydrate categories, such as:

- **Lower Carb:** Salad greens

- **Moderate Carb:** Cauliflower or summer squash

- **Higher Carb:** Broccoli or peppers

This lit will introduce the Green servings that you still need to consume while following this Diet Plan. These include all kinds of vegetables that have been categorized from lower, moderate, and high in terms of carbohydrate content. One serving of vegetables should be ½ cup unless otherwise specified.

Lower Carbohydrate: These are vegetables that contain low amounts of carbohydrates. If you are following the 5&1 Low Carb Diet Plan, then these vegetables are good for you.

A cup of green leafy vegetables, such as collard greens (raw), lettuce (green leaf, iceberg, butterhead, and romaine), spinach (raw), mustard greens, spring mix, bok choy (raw), and watercress.

½ cup of vegetables, including cucumbers, celery, radishes, white mushroom, sprouts (mung bean, alfalfa), arugula, turnip greens, escarole, nopales, Swiss chard (raw), jalapeño, and bok choy (cooked).

Moderate Carbohydrate: These are vegetables that contain moderate amounts of carbohydrates. Below are the types of vegetables that can be consumed in moderation:

½ cup of any vegetables such as asparagus, cauliflower, a fennel bulb, eggplant, portabella mushrooms, kale, cooked spinach, summer squash (zucchini and scallop).

Higher Carbohydrates: Foods that are under this category contain a high amount of starch. Make sure to consume limited amounts of these vegetables.

½ cup of the following: chayote squash, red cabbage, broccoli, cooked collard and mustard greens, green or wax beans, kohlrabi, kabocha squash, cooked leeks, any peppers, okra, raw scallion, summer squash such as straight neck and crookneck, tomatoes, spaghetti squash, turnips, jicama, cooked Swiss chard, and hearts of palm.

Low-Fat Dairy, Fresh Fruits and Whole Grains

Once users have attained the weight loss they wish through meal substitutes, lean protein, and non-starchy veggies; they can move on to a diet to preserve their weight.

On Low Carb's weight preservation plans, customers can start to reintroduce additional food groups. Low-fat dairy, fresh fruits, and whole grains are all included in Low Carb's "3&3" and "4&2&1" weight preservation programs

Non-Compliant Foods

Most carbohydrate-containing beverages and foods are forbidden while following the 5&1 diet plan. Certain fats, as well as all fried foods, are also not allowed because they are high in saturated fats.

There are many types of foods that are not allowed for the Low Carb Lean and Green Diet Plan. These foods either contain high amounts of fats or carbohydrates that can contribute to weight gain. Below are the types of foods that are not allowed under this particular diet—unless included in the Fuelings.

Generous Desserts

Unsurprisingly, this diet plan rejects spoiling your sugar desires with sweets like ice cream, cakes, cookies, and the likes.

Nevertheless, after the preliminary weight loss phase, reasonable sweet indulgences like freshly picked fruits or sweetened yogurt can be allowed their way back to your strict Low Carb diet.

High Caloric Additions

Shortening, butter, and elevated fat salad dressings increase flavor; however, they also increase large sums of calories. On Low Carb, you will be advised to keep additives to a minimum or substitute them for lesser calorie forms.

Alcohol

The Low Carb Lean and Green diet boosts customers to minimize alcohol consumption. If you are trying to stay within a stern calorie range, a 5-ounce glass of beer for 120 calories or the 150 calories in a 12-ounce glass of wine will add up fast.

Additionally, you cannot eat:

- **Fried Foods:** Meats, fish, shellfish, vegetables, sweets like pastries

- **Certain Fats:** Butter, coconut oil, solid shortening

- **Whole Fat Dairy:** Milk, cheese, yogurt

- **Alcohol:** all varieties

- **Sugar-Sweetened Beverages:** soda, fruit juice, sports drinks, energy drinks, sweet tea

The following foods will not be allowed while on the 5&1 Plan but added back through the 6-week transition phase and allowed during the 3&3 Plan:

- **Fruit:** All fresh fruit

- **Low in Fat or Fat-Free Dairy Products**: Milk, cheese, yogurt

- **Total grains:** Total grain bread, high roughage breakfast cereal, brown or black or red rice, total wheat pasta

- **Legumes:** Lentils, soybeans, peas, beans

- **Starchy Vegetables:** sweet potatoes, white potatoes, corn, peas

During the transition phase and 3&3 Plan, you are especially stimulated to consume berries over any other fruits, as they are lower in carbohydrates.

Chapter 3: How It Works

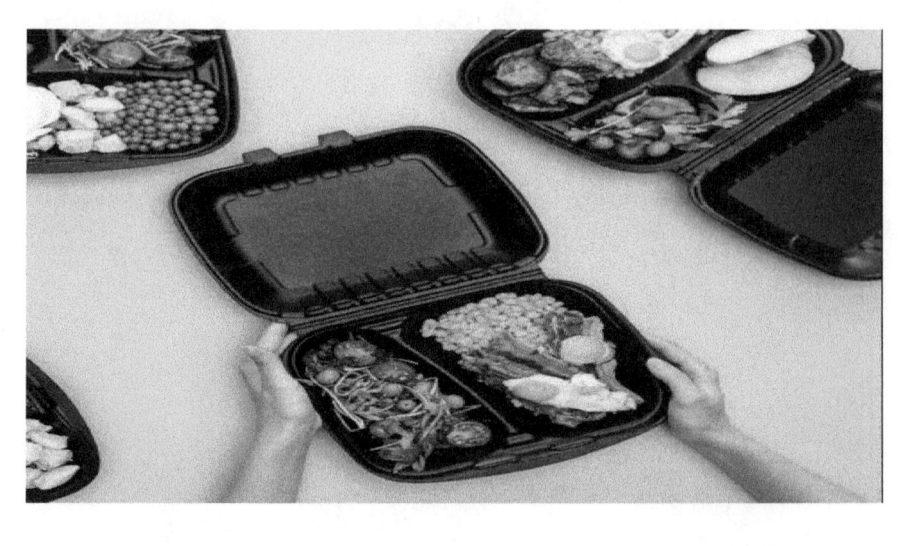

The Low Carb Lean and Green diet is viewed as a high-protein diet, with its protein having 10–35% of your daily calories. Be that as it may, the handled, powdered kind can prompt some not exactly beautiful outcomes. "The protein confines in addition to added substances can cause you to feel enlarged and have caused some undesirable GI symptoms, making better you off with unsweetened Greek yogurt for protein in a single smoothie,"—London says.

The FDA also doesn't direct dietary enhancements like shakes and powders for security and viability in a similar way it accomplishes food. "Powders and protein 'mixes' may have unwanted fixings, or could interface with a drug you might be taking," London includes, "making it extra critical to ensure your doctor knows about you attempting the arrangement."

How Nutritious Is the Low Carb Lean & Green Diet?

Below is the breakdown comparison of meals' nutritional content on the Optimal Weight 5&1 Plan and the federal government's 2015 Dietary Guidelines for Americans.

	Optimal Weight 5&1 Plan	Federal Government Recommendation
Calories	800–1000	Men 19–25: 2,800 26–45: 2,800 46–65: 2,400 65+: 2,200 Women 19–25: 2,200 26–50: 2,000

		51+: 1,800
Total fat **% of Calorie Intake**	20%	20–35%
Total Carbohydrates **% of Calorie Intake**	40%	45–65%
Sugars	10–20%	N/A
Fiber	25–30 g	Men 19–30: 34 g 31–50: 31 g 51+: 28 g Women 19–30: 28 g 31–50: 25 g

		51+: 22 g
Protein	40%	10–35%"
Sodium	Under 2,300 mg	Under 2,300 mg
Potassium	Average 3,000 mg	At least 4,700 mg
Calcium	1,000–1,200 mg	Men 1,000 mg Women 10–50: 1,000 mg 51+: 1,200 mg

Chapter 4: The Benefits and Disadvantages of the Low Carb Lean & Green Diet

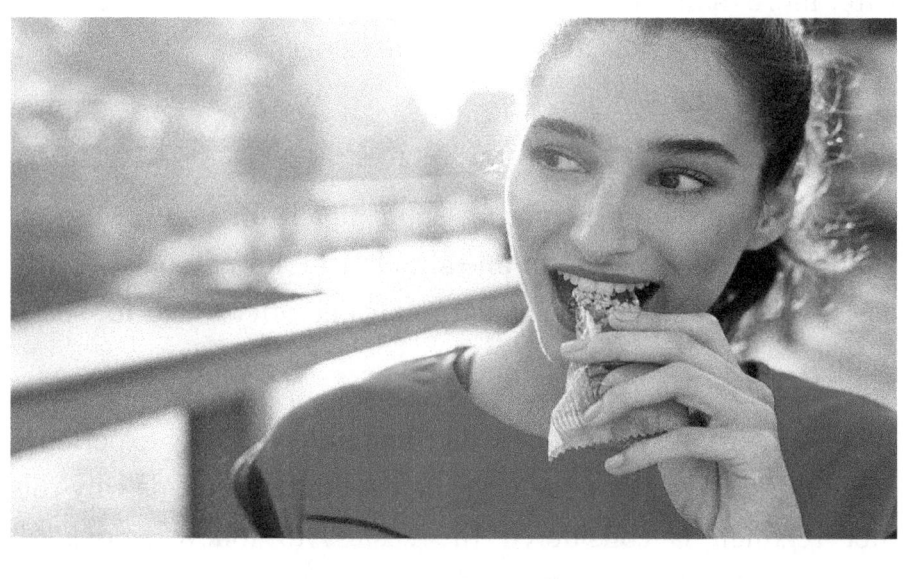

The Low Carb diet depends on restrictive dinner substitution items and careful, calorie-controlled arranged suppers, so there's very little space for change.

The 5&1 Plan limits calories to as low as 800–1000 every day, so it's not appropriate for individuals who are pregnant or practice intense physical exercises.

Extraordinary calorie limitation can cause exhaustion, mind haze, cerebral pains, or menstrual changes. Al things considered, the 5&1 alternative ought not to be utilized long haul.

Be that as it may, the 3&3, and 4&2&1 Plans are normally between 1100 and 2500 calories for every day and can gracefully be fitted to use for a more extended period

After more than my 1-year journey in doing Low Carb Diet, these are the following pros and cons I have noticed:

Pros

Low Carb's program may be a solid match for you on the off chance that you need a clear and simple-to-follow diet plan; it will assist you with getting in shape rapidly and offer words for social help.

When embarking on any new diet regimen, you may experience some difficulties along the way. Below are the reasons why this diet regimen is considered the easiest to follow among all commercial diet regimens.

Accomplishes rapid weight loss: Most solid individuals require around 1600 to 3000 calories each day to keep up their weight. Limiting that number to as low as 800 basically ensures weight loss for many people.

Low Carb's 5&1 Plan is intended for brisk weight loss, making it a strong choice for somebody with a clinical motivation to shed pounds quickly.

Easy to follow: As your diet depends on generally very quick and easy meals you won't have a hard time following the 5&1 plan.

Although you are encouraged to make 1 to 3 Lean and Green foods a day, contingent on the strategy, they are very simple to make—because the program will include detailed recipes and a list of food options for you to choose from.

It's not a ketogenic diet: Carbs are allowed and higher than the majority of weight-loss diets out there, just not refined ones.

No counting calories: You don't really need to count your calories when following this type of diet, just as long as you stick to the rule of Fuelings, meals, snacks, and water intake depending on your preference, may it be 5&1, 4&2&1 or 3&3.

Cons

It's tough the first weeks: You may feel hungry, but it will fade away in the next few weeks

Calories are lower than what is suggested in a long-term diet: Even though the Low Carb's diet plan emphasizes frequently eating throughout the day, each of its "Fuelings" only provides 110 calories. "Lean and Green" meals are also low in calories.

When you are eating fewer calories in general, you may find the plan leaves you hungry and unsatisfied. You may also feel more easily fatigued and irritable.

Weight loss might be impractical: One test recognizable to anybody on a careful nutritional plan is deciding how to keep up weight loss once they've finished the program.

The equivalent goes for Low Carb's program. At the point when clients return to eating ordinary suppers rather than the plan's dinner substitutions, they may find that the weight they lost is immediately recovered.

Calorie limitation may leave you eager or exhausted: Although Low Carb's diet plan accentuates eating much of the time for the day, every one of its "Fuelings" just gives 110 calories. "Lean and green" suppers are additionally low in calories.

At the point when you're eating fewer calories, by and large, you may discover the plan leaves you ravenous and unsatisfied. You may likewise feel all the more effectively exhausted and even crabby.

Eating times can get exhausting or feel disengaging: Low Carb's dependence on feast supplanting can meddle with the social parts of getting ready and eating food.

Clients may think that it's ungainly or disillusioning to have a shake or soup at family supper time or when feasting out with peers.

Chapter 5: A Deeper Look into the Low Carb Lean & Green Diet

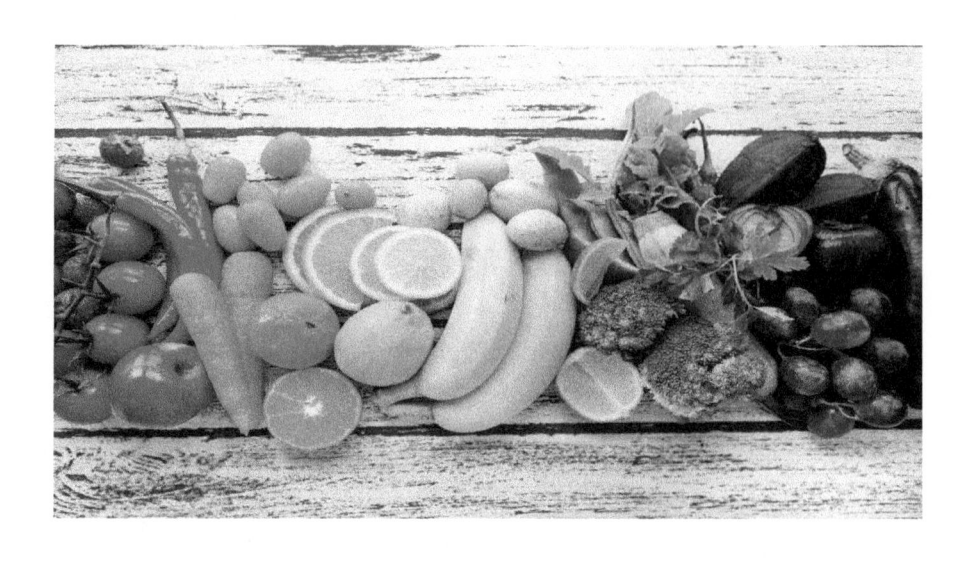

Beginning Phase

Most people begin with the Optimal Weight 5&1 weight loss program, which is an 800–1,000 calorie routine said to help you lose 12 pounds over 12 weeks (5.4 kg). You consume 5 Fuelings meals every day on this menu and 1 Lean and Green meal. You're expected to consume one meal every 2–3 hours and, on most days of the week, involve 30 minutes of a moderate workout. In sum, the Fuelings and food focus on providing no more than 100 grams of carbohydrates per day.

The aim of Lean and Green meals is to be rich in proteins and lighter in carbs. One meal contains 5–7 ounces of cooked lean protein (145–200 grams), three pieces of veggies, and up to 2 portions of good fats.

This schedule also involves one extra snack a day. Three veggie sticks, 1/2 cup (60 grams) of sugar-free jelly, or 1/2 ounce (14 grams) of nuts are Plan-approved snacks. A dining-out guide that describes how to eat a Lean and Green meal at any favorite place is also included in the program. Please remember that the 5&1 Program actively prohibits alcohol.

Maintenance Phase

You begin a six-week maintenance period after you hit the target weight, which includes steadily raising calories of not more than 1,550 calories a day and incorporating a wider wide variety of foods, like whole grains, vegetables, and low-fat dairy goods. You are expected to switch over to the Low Carb 3&3 plan after six weeks, which involves 3 Lean and Green meals and 3 Fuelings every day, plus regular training.

The following are all the foods that are allowed to prepare your Lean & Green meals at home. They include:

- Healthy fats (canola oil, avocado, low-carb salad dressing, olive oil, and olive leaves, etc.)

- Shellfish (crab, shrimp, scallops)

- Whole eggs (maximum three per week)

- turkey or Chicken

- Ground meat (at least 85 percent lean)

- Fish (cod, tuna, tilapia, flounder)

- Egg Beaters or Egg whites

- Tenderloin or Porkchop

- Game meat (buffalo)

- Tofu

- Lean beef

- Vegetables (leafy greens, radishes, cucumbers, mushrooms, asparagus, and broccoli, etc.)

The diet recommends a reduction in the consumption of caffeine or soda afternoon per day as it comes to beverages

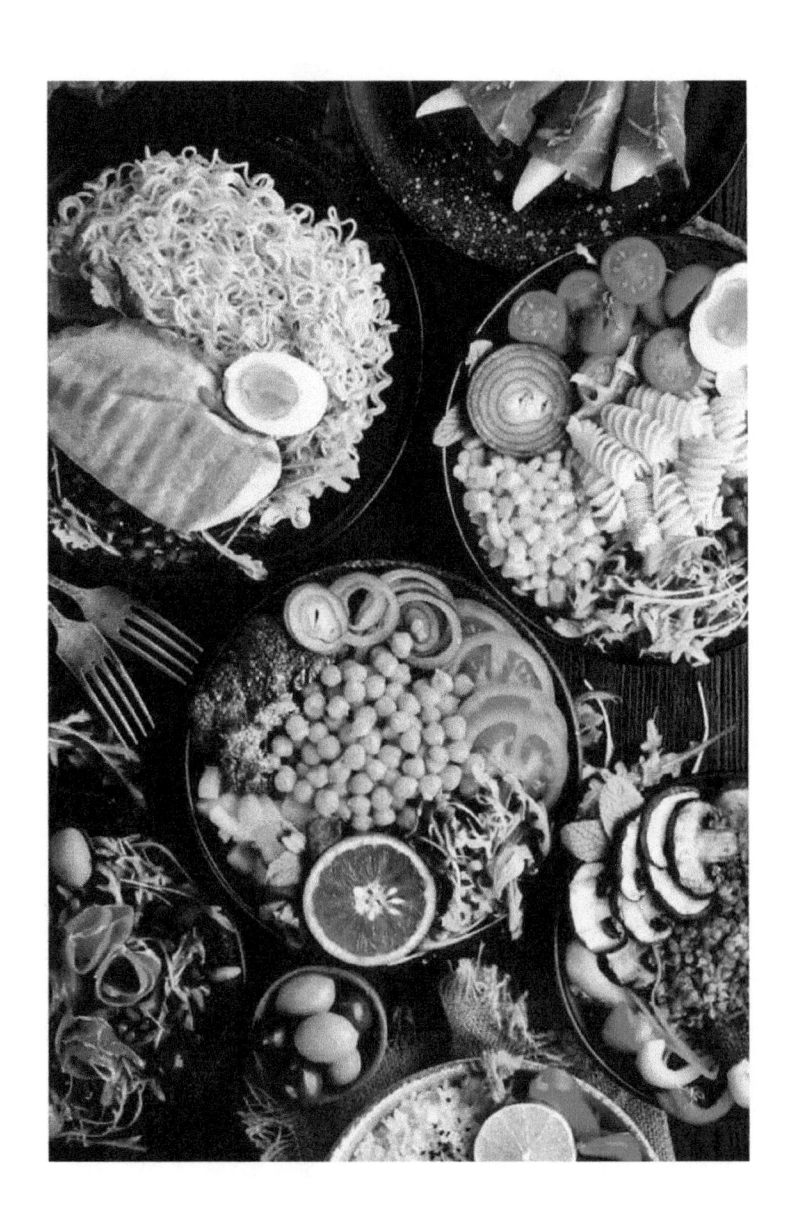

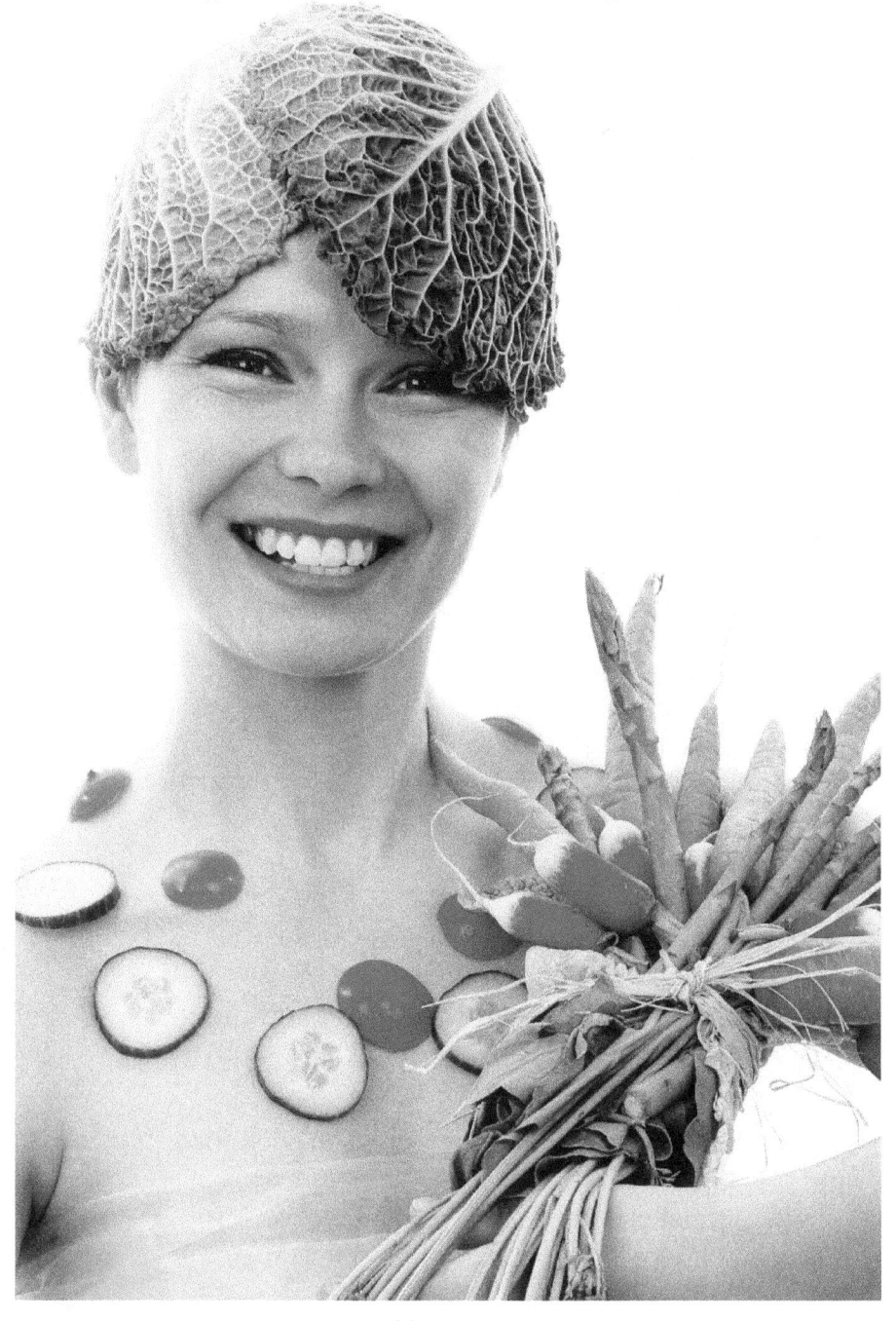

1. Moules Marinieres

Preparation Time: 10 minutes

Cooking Time: 30 minutes

Servings: 4

Ingredients:

- 2 tbsp. unsalted butter

- 1 leek

- 1 shallot

- 2 garlic cloves

- 2 bay leaves

- 1 cup white wine

- 2 lb. mussels

- 2 tbsp. mayonnaise

- 1 tbsp. lemon zest

- 2 tbsp. parsley

- 1 sourdough bread

Directions:

1. In a saucepan, melt the butter, add the leeks, garlic, bay leaves, shallot, and cook until vegetables are soft.

2. Bring to a boil, add mussels, and cook for 1–2 minutes.

3. Transfer mussels to a bowl and cover.

4. Whisk in the remaining butter with mayonnaise and return mussels to the pot.

5. Add the lemon juice, parsley lemon zest, and stir to combine.

Nutrition:

- Calories: 321
- Carbs: 2 g
- Cholesterol: 13 mg
- Fats: 17 g

- Fiber: 2 g
- Protein: 9 g
- Sodium: 312 mg

2. Steamed Mussels with Coconut-Curry

Preparation Time: 15 minutes

Cooking Time: 20 minutes

Servings: 4

Ingredients:

- 6 sprigs cilantro

- 2 garlic cloves

- 2 shallots

- ¼ tsp. coriander seeds

- ¼ tsp. red chili flakes

- 1 tsp. zest

- 1 can coconut milk

- 1 tbsp. vegetable oil

- 1 tbsp. curry paste

- 1 tbsp. brown sugar

- 1 tbsp. fish sauce

- 2 lb. mussels

Directions:

1. In a bowl, combine the lime zest, cilantro stems, shallot, garlic, coriander seed, chili, and salt.

2. In a saucepan, heat oil, add the garlic, shallots, pounded paste, and curry paste.

3. Cook for 3–4 minutes. Add the coconut milk, sugar, and fish sauce.

4. Bring to a simmer and add the mussels.

5. Stir in the lime juice, cilantro leaves, and cook for a couple more minutes.

6. When ready, remove from heat and serve.

Nutrition:

- Calories: 209

- Carbs: 6 g

- Cholesterol: 13 mg

- Fats: 7 g

- Fiber: 2 g

- Protein: 17 g

- Sodium: 193 mg

3. Tuna Noodle Casserole

Preparation Time: 15 minutes

Cooking Time: 20 minutes

Servings: 4

Ingredients:

- 2 oz. egg noodles
- 4 oz. fraiche
- 1 egg
- 1 tsp. cornstarch
- 1 tbsp. juice from 1 lemon
- 1 can tuna
- 1 cup peas
- ¼ cup parsley

Directions:

1. Place noodles in a saucepan with water and bring to a boil.

2. In a bowl, combine the egg, crème fraîche, and lemon juice, whisk well.

3. When noodles are cooked, add crème fraîche mixture to skillet and mix well.

4. Add the tuna, peas, parsley lemon juice, and mix well.

5. When ready, remove from heat and serve.

Nutrition:

- Calories: 214
- Carbs: 2 g
- Cholesterol: 73 mg
- Fats: 7 g

- Fiber: 2 g
- Protein: 19 g
- Sodium: 308 g

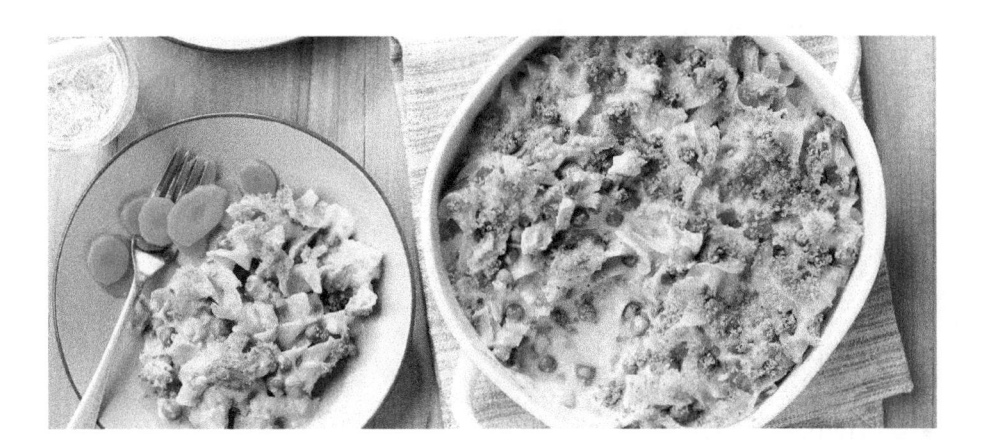

4. Salmon Burgers

Preparation Time: 10 minutes

Cooking Time: 15 minutes

Servings: 4

Ingredients:

- 1 lb. salmon fillets

- 1 onion

- ¼ dill fronds

- 1 tbsp. honey

- 1 tbsp. horseradish

- 1 tbsp. mustard

- 1 tbsp. olive oil

- 2 toasted split rolls

- 1 avocado

Directions:

1. Place salmon fillets in a blender and blend until smooth, transfer to a bowl, add the onion, dill, honey, and horseradish, and mix well.

2. Season with salt and pepper and form 4 patties.

3. In a bowl, combine the mustard, honey, mayonnaise, and dill.

4. In a skillet, heat oil, add salmon patties, and cook for 2–3 minutes each side.

5. When ready, remove from heat.

6. Divide the lettuce and onion between the buns.

7. Place salmon patty on top and spoon mustard mixture and avocado slices.

8. Serve when ready.

Nutrition:

- Calories: 189

- Carbs: 6 g

- Cholesterol: 3 mg

- Fats: 7 g

- Fiber: 4 g

- Protein: 12 g

- Sodium: 293 mg

5. Seared Scallops

Preparation Time: 15 minutes

Cooking Time: 20 minutes

Servings: 4

Ingredients:

- 1 lb. sea scallops

- 1 tbsp. canola oil

Directions:

1. Season scallops and refrigerate for a couple of minutes.

2. In a skillet, heat the oil, add scallops and cook for 1–2 minutes each side.

3. When ready, remove from heat and serve.

Nutrition:

- Calories 283

- Carbs: 10 g
- Fiber: 2 g

- Cholesterol: 3 mg
- Protein: 9 g

- Fats: 8 g
- Sodium: 271 mg

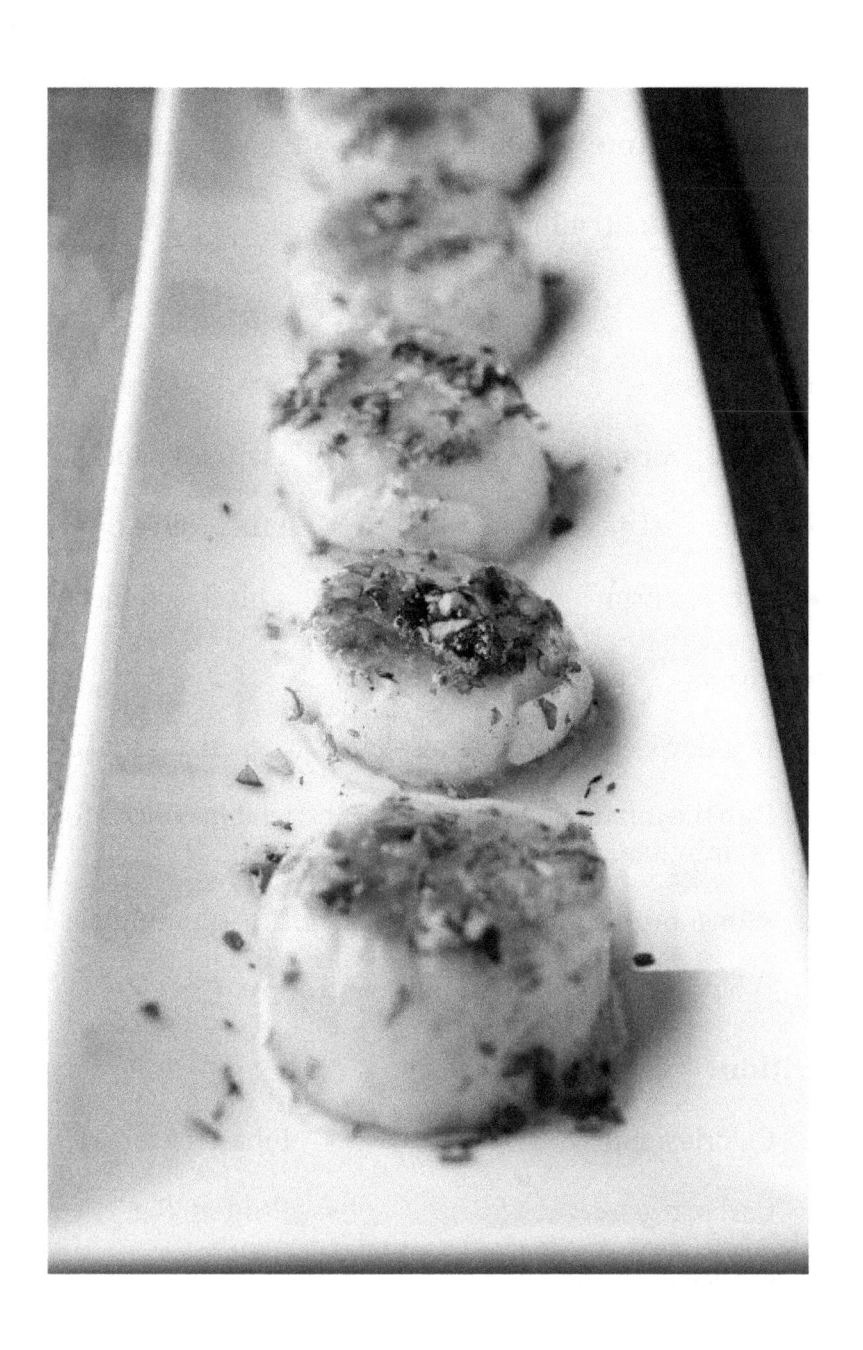

6. Black Cod

Preparation Time: 15 minutes

Cooking Time: 20 minutes

Servings: 4

Ingredients:

- ¼ cup miso paste
- ¼ cup sake
- 1 tbsp. mirin
- 1 tsp. soy sauce
- 1 tbsp. olive oil
- 4 black cod filets

Directions:

1. In a bowl, combine the miso, soy sauce, oil, and sake.

2. Rub the mixture over cod fillets and let it marinade for 20–30 minutes.

3. Adjust broiler and broil cod filets for 10–12 minutes.

4. When fish is cooked, remove, and serve.

Nutrition:

- Calories: 231
- Carbs: 2 g
- Cholesterol: 13 mg
- Fats: 15 g
- Fiber: 2 g
- Protein: 8 g
- Sodium: 298 mg

7. Miso-Glazed Salmon

Preparation Time: 10 minutes

Cooking Time: 40 minutes

Servings: 4

Ingredients:

- ¼ cup red miso
- ¼ cup sake
- 1 tbsp. soy sauce
- 1 tbsp. vegetable oil
- 4 salmon fillets

Directions:

1. In a bowl, combine the sake, oil, soy sauce, and miso.
2. Rub the mixture over salmon fillets and marinade for 20–30 minutes.
3. Preheat a broiler.
4. Broil the salmon fillets for 5–10 minutes.
5. When ready, remove, and serve.

Nutrition:

- Calories: 198
- Carbs: 5 g
- Cholesterol: 12 mg
- Fats: 10 g
- Fiber: 2 g
- Protein: 6 g
- Sodium: 257 mg

8. Arugula and Sweet Potato Salad

Preparation Time: 10 minutes

Cooking Time: 20 minutes

Servings: 4

Ingredients:

- 1 lb. sweet potatoes
- 1 cup walnuts
- 1 tbsp. olive oil
- 1 cup water
- 1 tbsp. soy sauce
- 3 cups arugula

Directions:

1. Bake potatoes at 400°F (204°C) until tender, remove and set aside.

2. In a bowl, drizzle walnuts with olive oil and microwave for 2–3 minutes or until toasted.

3. In a bowl, combine all the salad ingredients and mix well.

4. Pour over the soy sauce and serve.

Nutrition:

- Calories: 189
- Carbs: 2 g
- Cholesterol: 13 mg
- Fats: 7 g
- Fiber: 2 g
- Protein: 10 g
- Sodium: 301 mg

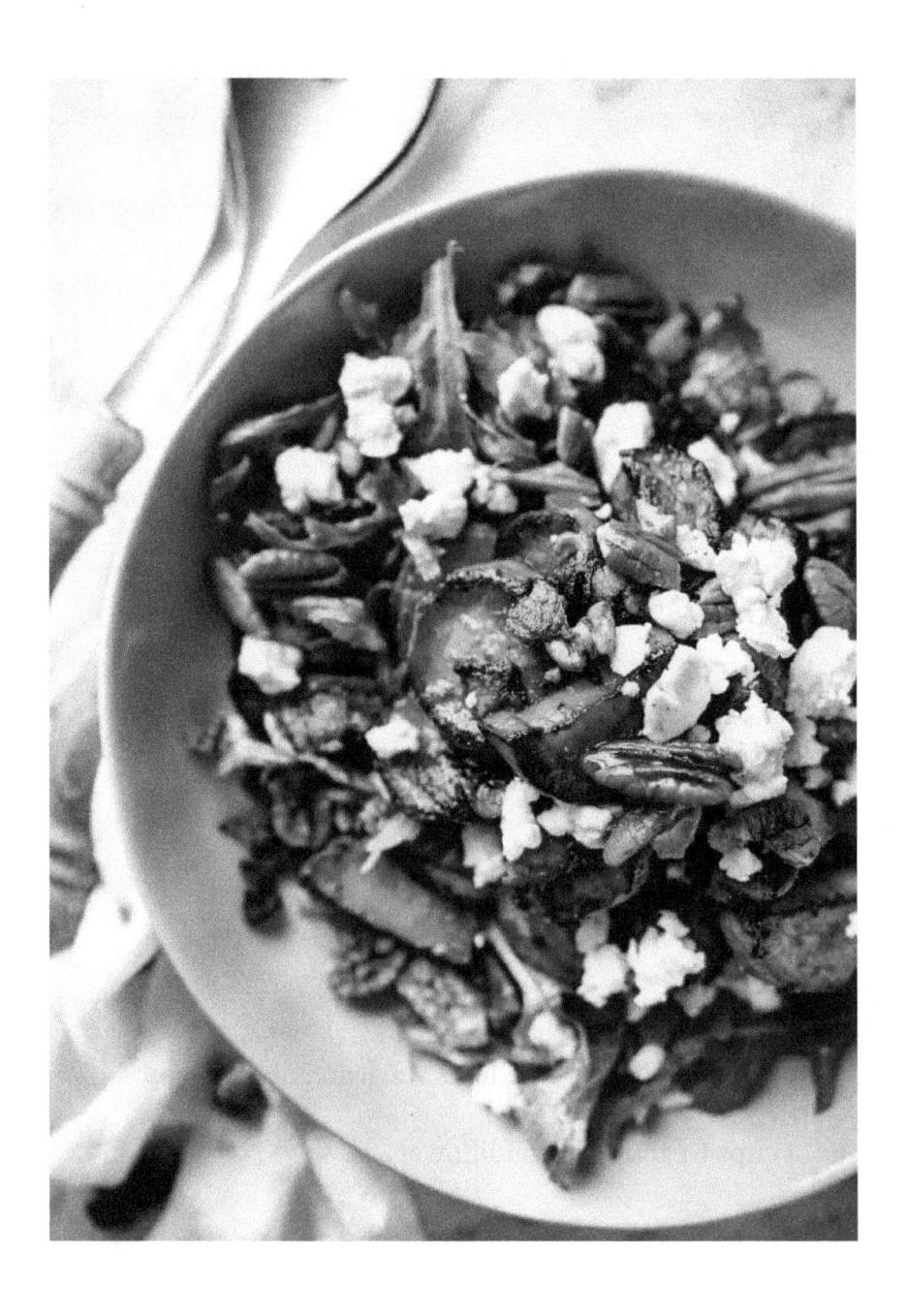

9. Instant Pot Chipotle Chicken & Cauliflower Rice Bowls

Preparation Time: 10 minutes

Cooking Time: 20 minutes

Servings: 4

Ingredients:

- 1/3 cup salsa

- 14.5 oz. can fire-roasted diced tomatoes

- 1 canned chipotle pepper + 1 tsp. sauce

- ½ tsp. dried oregano

- 1 tsp. cumin

- 1 ½ lb. b1 less, skinless chicken breast

- ¼ tsp. salt

- 1 cup reduced-fat shredded Mexican cheese blend

- 4 cups frozen riced cauliflower

- ½ medium-sized avocado, sliced

Directions:

1. Combine the first ingredients in a blender and blend until they become smooth.

2. Place chicken inside your instant pot, and pour the sauce over it. Cover the lid and close the pressure valve. Set it to 20 minutes at high temperature. Let the pressure release on its own before opening. Remove the piece and the chicken and then add it back to the sauce.

3. Microwave the riced cauliflower according to the directions on the package.

4. Before you serve, divide the riced cauliflower, cheese, avocado, and chicken equally among the 4 bowls.

Nutrition:

- Calories: 287

- Protein: 35 g

- Carbs: 19 g

- Fats: 12 g

10. Lemon Garlic Oregano Chicken with Asparagus

Preparation Time: 5 minutes

Cooking Time: 40 minutes

Servings: 4

Ingredients:

- 1 small lemon, juiced; this should be about 2 tbsp. lemon juice

- 1 ¾ lb. bone-in, skinless chicken thighs

- 2 tbsp. fresh oregano, minced

- 2 garlic cloves, minced

- 2 lbs. asparagus, trimmed

- ¼ tsp. each or less for black pepper and salt

Directions:

1. Preheat the oven to about 350°F (177°C).

2. Put the chicken in a medium-sized bowl. Now, add the garlic, oregano, lemon juice, pepper, and salt and toss together to combine.

3. Roast the chicken in the air fryer oven until it reaches an internal temperature of 165°F (74°C) in about 40 minutes. Once the chicken thighs have been cooked, remove and keep aside to rest.

4. Now, steam the asparagus on a stovetop or in a microwave to the desired doneness.

5. Serve asparagus with the roasted chicken thighs.

Nutrition:

- Calories: 350
- Carbs: 10 g
- Fats: 10 g
- Protein: 32 g

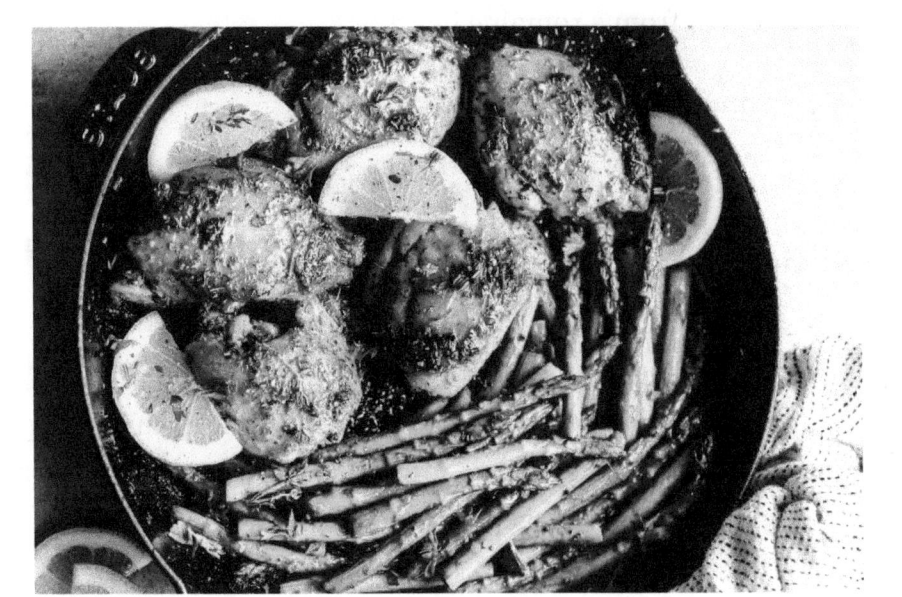

11. Sheet Pan Chicken Fajita Lettuce Wraps

Preparation Time: 15 minutes

Cooking Time: 30 minutes

Servings: 2

Ingredients:

- 1 lb. chicken breast, thinly sliced into strips

- 2 tsp. olive oil

- 2 bell peppers, thinly sliced into strips

- 2 tsp. fajita seasoning

- 6 leaves from a romaine heart

- ½ lime juice

- ¼ cup plain of non-Fat Greek yogurt

Directions:

1. Preheat your oven to about 400°F (204°C).

2. Combine all of the ingredients except for lettuce in a large plastic bag that can be resealed. Mix very well to coat vegetables and chicken with oil and seasoning evenly.

3. Spread the contents of the bag evenly on a foil-lined baking sheet. Bake it for about 25–30 minutes, until the chicken is thoroughly cooked.

4. Serve on lettuce leaves and top with Greek yogurt if you like.

Nutrition:

- Calories: 387
- Fats: 6 g
- Carbs: 14 g
- Protein: 18 g

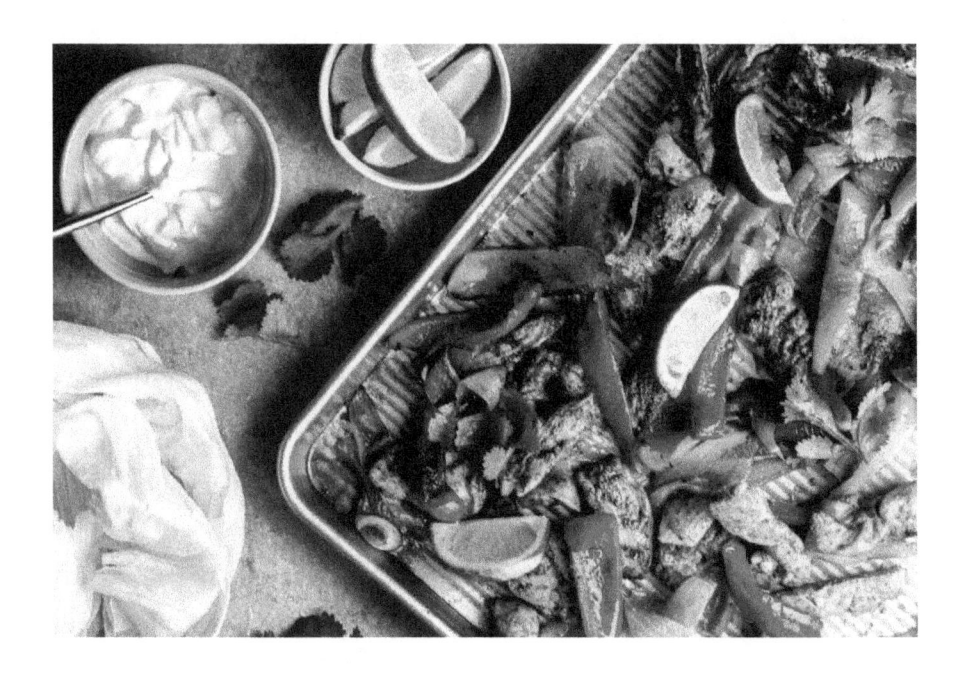

12. Savory Cilantro Salmon

Preparation Time: 10 minutes

Cooking Time: 30 minutes

Servings: 4

Ingredients:

- 2 tbsp. fresh lime or lemon
- 4 cups fresh cilantro, divided
- 2 tbsp. hot red pepper sauce
- ½ tsp. salt. Divided
- 1 tsp. cumin
- 4, 7 oz. salmon filets
- ½ cup (4 oz.) water
- 2 cups sliced red bell pepper
- 2 cups sliced yellow bell pepper
- 2 cups sliced green bell pepper
- Cooking spray
- ½ tsp. pepper

Directions:

1. Get a blender or food processor and combine half of the cilantro, lime juice or lemon, cumin, hot red pepper sauce,

water, and salt; then purée until they become smooth. Transfer the marinade into a large resealable plastic bag.

2. Add salmon to marinade. Seal the bag, squeeze out air that might have been trapped inside, turn it to coat salmon. Refrigerate for about 1 hour, turning as often as possible.

3. Now, after marinating, preheat your oven to about 400°F (204°C). Arrange the pepper slices in a single layer in a slightly-greased, medium-sized square baking dish. Bake it for 20 minutes, turn the pepper slices once.

4. Drain your salmon and do away with the marinade. Crust the upper part of the salmon with the remaining chopped, fresh cilantro. Place salmon on top of the pepper slices and bake for about 12–14 minutes until you observe that the fish flakes easily when it is being tested with a fork.

5. Enjoy!

Nutrition:

- Calories: 350
- Carbs: 15 g
- Protein: 42 g
- Fats: 13 g

13. Vegetables in air Fryer

Preparation Time: 20 minutes

Cooking Time: 30 minutes

Servings: 2

Ingredients:

- 2 potatoes
- 1 zucchini
- 1 onion
- 1 red pepper
- 1 green pepper

Directions:

1. Cut the potatoes into slices.

2. Cut the onion into rings.

3. Cut the zucchini into slices.

4. Cut the peppers into strips.

5. Put all the ingredients in a bowl and add a little salt, ground pepper, and some extra virgin olive oil.

6. Mix well.

7. Pass to the basket of the air fryer.

8. Select 160°F (71°C) and 30 minutes.

9. Check that the vegetables are up to your taste.

Nutrition:

- Calories: 135
- Protein: 4 g
- Carbs: 2 g
- Fiber: 5 g
- Fats: 11 g

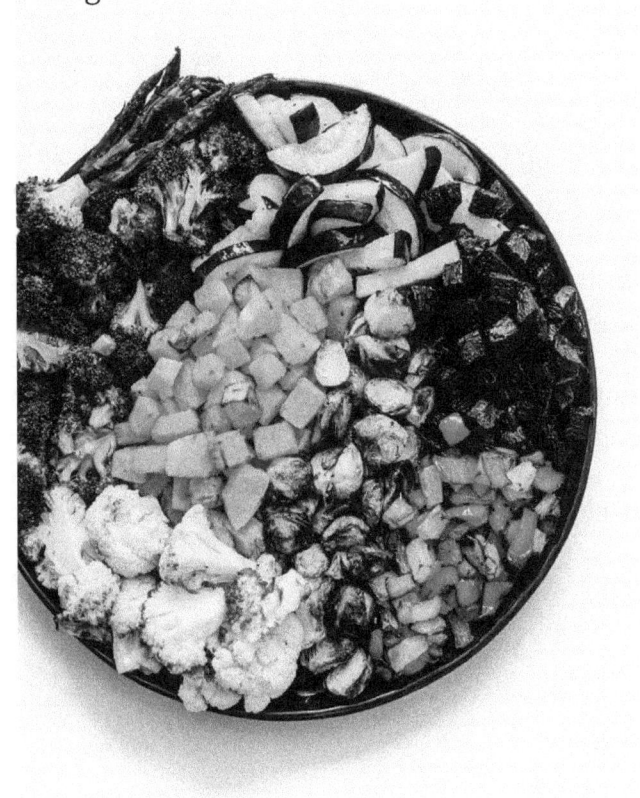

14. Crispy Rye Bread Snacks with Guacamole and Anchovies

Preparation Time: 10 minutes

Cooking Time: 10 minutes

Servings: 4

Ingredients:

- 4 slices rye bread
- Guacamole
- Anchovies in oil

Directions:

1. Cut each slice of bread into 3 strips.

2. Place in the basket of the air fryer, without piling up, and go in batches giving it the touch you want to give it. You can select 180°F (82°C) and 10 minutes.

3. When you have all the crusty rye bread strips, put a layer of guacamole on top, whether homemade or commercial.

4. In each bread, place 2 anchovies on the guacamole.

Nutrition:

- Calories: 180
- Protein: 4 g
- Carbs: 4 g
- Fiber: 9 g
- Fats: 11 g

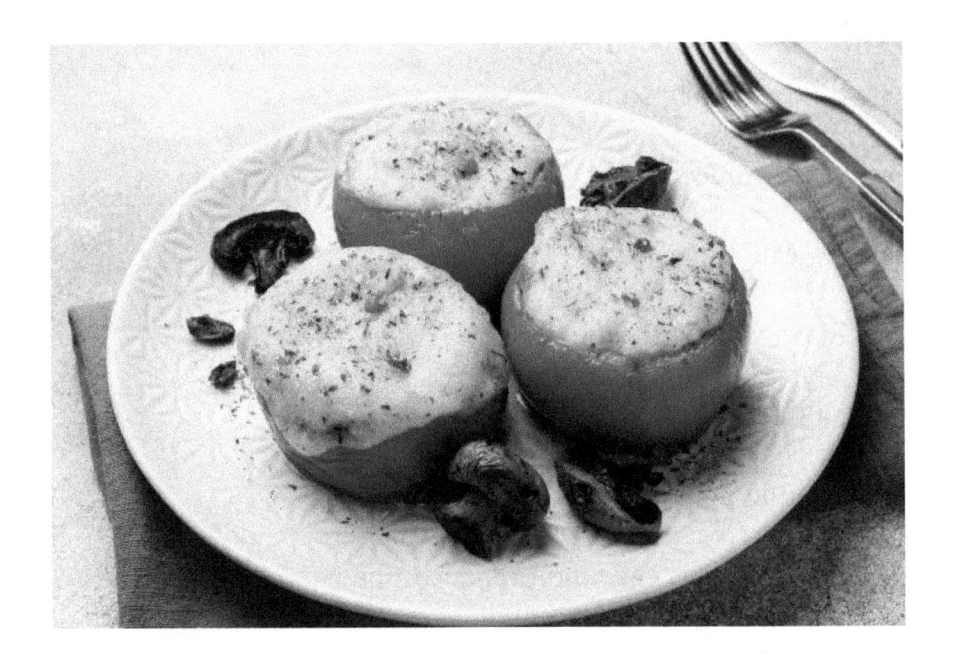

15. Mushrooms Stuffed with Tomato

Preparation Time: 5 minutes

Cooking Time: 50 minutes

Servings: 4

Ingredients:

- 8 large mushrooms

- 250 g minced meat

- 4 garlic cloves

- Extra virgin olive oil

- Salt

- Ground pepper

- Flour, beaten egg, and breadcrumbs

- Frying oil

- Fried tomato sauce

Directions:

1. Remove the stem from the mushrooms and chop it. Peel the garlic and chop it. Put some extra virgin olive oil in a pan and add the garlic and mushroom stems.

72

2. Sauté and add minced meat. Sauté well until the meat is well cooked and seasoned.

3. Fill the mushrooms with the minced meat.

4. Press well and take it into the freezer and leave it for 30 minutes.

5. Pass the mushrooms with flour, beaten egg, and breadcrumbs.

6. Place the mushrooms in the basket of the air fryer.

7. Select 20 minutes, 180°F (82°C).

8. Once cooked, distribute the mushrooms in the dishes.

9. Heat the tomato sauce and cover the stuffed mushrooms.

Nutrition:

- Calories: 160

- Carbs: 2 g

- Fats: 11 g

- Protein: 4 g

- Fiber: 0 g

16. Fennel and Arugula Salad with Fig Vinaigrette

Preparation Time: 15 minutes

Cooking Time: 10 minutes

Servings: 6

Ingredients:

- 5 oz. washed and dried arugula

- 1 small fennel bulb, it can be either shaved or tiny sliced.

- 2 tbsp. extra virgin oil or any cooking oil

- 1 tsp. lemon zest

- ½ tsp. salt

- Pepper (freshly ground)

- Pecorino

Directions:

1. Mix the arugula and shaved funnel in a serving bowl.

2. On another bowl, mix the olive oil or cooking oil, lemon zest, salt, and pepper.

3. Shake together until it becomes creamy and smooth.

4. Pour and dress over the salad, tossing gently for it to combine.

5. Peel or shave out some pecorino slices and put them on top of the salad.

6. Serve immediately.

Nutrition:

- Protein: 2.1 g
- Carbs: 14.3 g
- Dietary Fiber: 3.4 g
- Sugars: 9.1 g
- Fats: 9.7 g

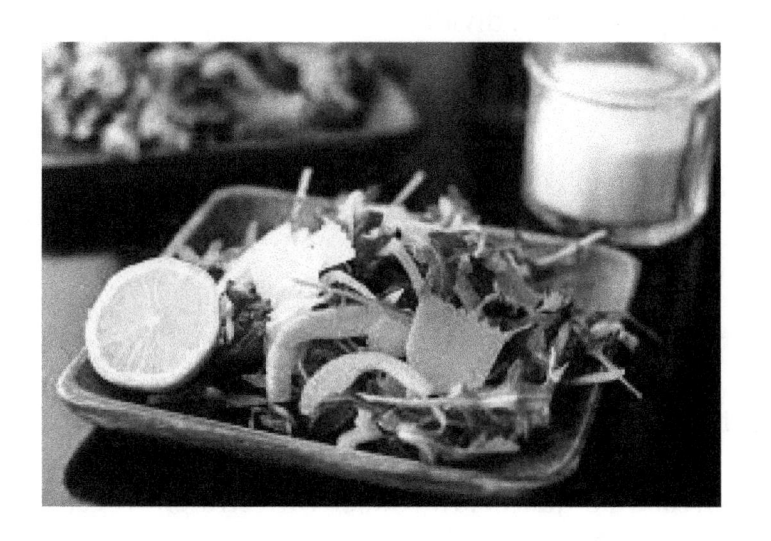

17. Mixed Potato Gratin

Preparation Time: 20 minutes

Cooking Time: 7 to 9 hours

Servings: 8

Ingredients:

- 6 Yukon Gold potatoes, thinly sliced

- 3 sweet potatoes, peeled and thinly sliced

- 2 onions, thinly sliced

- 4 garlic cloves, minced

- 3 tbsp. whole-wheat flour

- 4 cups 2% milk, divided

- 1½ cups roasted vegetable broth

- 3 tbsp. melted butter

- 1 tsp. dried thyme leaves

- 1½ cups shredded Havarti cheese

Directions:

1. Grease a 6-quart slow cooker with straight vegetable oil.

2. In the slow cooker, layer the potatoes, onions, and garlic.

3. In a large bowl, mix the flour with ½ cup the milk until well combined.

4. Gradually add the remaining milk, stirring with a wire whisk to avoid lumps.

5. Stir in the vegetable broth, melted butter, and thyme leaves.

6. Pour the milk mixture over the potatoes in the slow cooker and top with the cheese.

7. Cover and cook over low heat for 7 to 9 hours, or until the potatoes are tender when pierced with a fork.

Nutrition:

- Calories: 415
- Carbs: 42 g
- Sugar: 10 g
- Fiber: 3 g
- Fats: 22 g
- Saturated Fats: 13 g
- Protein: 17 g
- Sodium: 431 mg

18. Green Pea Guacamole

Preparation Time: 15 minutes

Cooking Time: 35 minutes

Servings: 4

Ingredients:

- 1 tsp. crushed garlic

- 1 chopped tomato

- 3 cups frozen green peas, chopped

- 5 green chopped onions

- 1/6 tsp. hot sauce

- ½ tsp. grounded cumin

- ½ cup lime juice

Directions:

1. Blend the peas, garlic, lime juice and cumin until it is smoothened.

2. Stir the tomatoes, green onion and hot sauce into the mixture.

3. Then, add salt to taste.

4. Cover it and put it into the refrigerator for a minimum of 30 minutes.

5. This will allow the flavors to blend very well.

Nutrition:

- Calories: 40.7
- Fats: 0.2 g
- Cholesterol: 0.0 mg
- Sodium: 157.4 mg
- Carbs: 7.6 g
- Dietary Fiber: 1.7 g
- Protein: 2.7 g

19. Salmon Florentine

Preparation Time: 5 minutes

Cooking Time: 30 minutes

Servings: 4

Ingredients:

- 1 ½ cups chopped cherry tomatoes

- ½ cup chopped green onions

- 2 garlic cloves, minced

- 1 tsp. olive oil

- 12 oz. package frozen chopped spinach, thawed and patted dry

- ¼ tsp. crushed red pepper flakes

- ½ cup part-skim ricotta cheese

- ¼ tsp. each for pepper and salt

- 4 (5 ½ oz.) wild salmon fillets

- Cooking spray

Directions:

1. Preheat the oven to 350°F (177°C).

2. Get a medium skillet to cook onions in oil until they start to soften, which should be in about 2 minutes. You can then add garlic inside the skillet and cook for an extra 1 minute. Add the spinach, red pepper flakes, tomatoes, pepper, and salt. Cook for 2 minutes while stirring. Remove the pan from the heat and let it cool for about 10 minutes. Stir in the ricotta.

3. Put a quarter of the spinach mixture on top of each salmon fillet. Place the fillets on a slightly-greased rimmed baking sheet and bake them for 15 minutes or until you are sure that the salmon has been thoroughly cooked.

Nutrition:

- Calories: 350

- Carbs: 15 g

- Protein: 42 g

- Fats: 13 g

20. Tomato Braised Cauliflower with Chicken

Preparation Time: 10 minutes

Cooking Time: 30 minutes

Servings: 4

Ingredients:

- 4 garlic cloves, sliced

- 3 scallions, to be trimmed and cut into 1-inch pieces

- ¼ tsp. dried oregano

- ¼ tsp. crushed red pepper flakes

- 4 ½ cups cauliflower

- 1 ½ cups diced canned tomatoes

- 1 cup fresh basil, gently torn

- ½ tsp. each of pepper and salt, divided

- 1 ½ tsp. olive oil

- 1 ½ lb. boneless, skinless chicken breasts

Directions:

1. Get a saucepan and combine the garlic, scallions, oregano, crushed red pepper, cauliflower, and tomato, and add ¼ cup water. Get everything boiling together and add ¼ tsp. of and salt for seasoning, then cover the pot with a lid. Let it simmer for 10 minutes and stir as often as possible until you observe that the cauliflower is tender. Now, wrap up the seasoning with the remaining ¼ tsp. pepper and salt.

2. Toss the chicken breast with oil (olive preferably), and let it roast in the oven at 450°F (232°C) for 20 minutes and an internal temperature of 165°F (74°C). Allow the chicken to rest for like 10 minutes.

3. Now slice the chicken, and serve on a bed of tomato braised cauliflower.

Nutrition:

- Calories: 290

- Fats: 10 g

- Carbs: 13 g

- Protein: 38 g

21. Cheeseburger Soup

Preparation Time: 20 minutes

Cooking Time: 25 minutes

Servings: 4

Ingredients:

- ¼ cup chopped onion

- 14.5 oz. can diced tomato

- 1 lb. 90% lean ground beef

- ¾ cup diced celery

- 2 tsp. Worcestershire sauce

- 3 cups low sodium chicken broth

- ¼ tsp. salt

- 1 tsp. dried parsley

- 7 cups baby spinach

- ¼ tsp. ground pepper

- 4 oz. reduced-Fat shredded cheddar cheese

Directions:

1. Get a large soup pot and cook the beef until it becomes brown. Add the celery and onion, sauté until it becomes tender. Remove from the fire and drain excess liquid.

2. Stir in the broth, tomatoes, parsley, Worcestershire sauce, pepper, and salt. Cover and allow it to simmer on low heat for about 20 minutes.

3. Add spinach and leave it to cook until it becomes wilted in about 1–3 minutes. Top each of your servings with 1 oz. cheese.

Nutrition:

- Calories: 400
- Carbs: 11 g
- Protein: 44 g
- Fats: 20 g

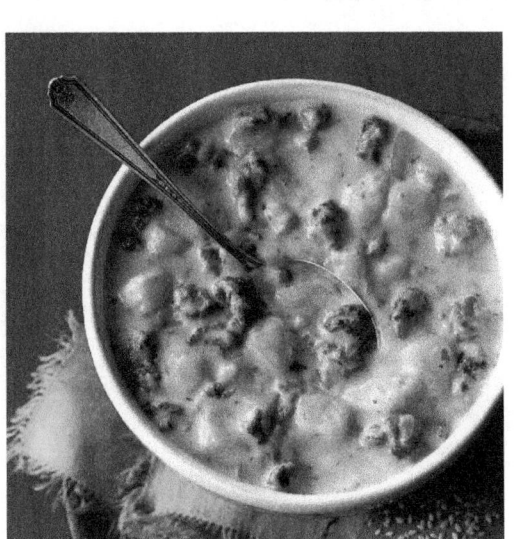

22. Braised Collard Greens in Peanut Sauce with Pork Tenderloin

Preparation Time: 20 minutes

Cooking Time: 1 hour 12 minutes

Servings: 4

Ingredients:

- 2 cups chicken stock

- 12 cups chopped collard greens

- 5 tbsp. powdered peanut butter

- 3 garlic cloves, crushed

- 1 tsp. salt

- ½ tsp. allspice

- ½ tsp. black pepper

- 2 tsp. lemon juice

- ¾ tsp. hot sauce

- 1 ½ lb. pork tenderloin

Directions:

1. Get a pot with a tight-fitting lid and combine the collards with the garlic, chicken stock, hot sauce, and half of the pepper and salt. Cook over low heat for about 1 hour or until the collards become tender.

2. Once the collards are tender, stir in the allspice, lemon juice, and powdered peanut butter. Keep warm.

3. Season the pork tenderloin with the remaining pepper and salt, and broil in a toaster oven for 10 minutes or when you have an internal temperature of 145°F (62°C). Make sure to turn the tenderloin every 2 minutes to achieve an even browning all over. After that, you can take away the pork from the oven and allow it to rest for like 5 minutes.

4. Slice the pork as you will.

Nutrition:

- Calories: 320

- Fats: 10 g

- Carbs: 15 g

- Protein: 45 g

23. Tomato Salad and Crunchy Cauliflower

Preparation Time: 15 minutes, **Additional Time:** 30 minutes

Cooking Time: 0

Servings: 6

Ingredients:

- 1 cup cherry tomatoes or more if desired, should be halved

- 2 garlic cloves (blanks), should be minced

- ¼ cup minced fresh parsley

- ¼ cup minced red onion

- 1 large head of cauliflower, should be chopped into pieces

- Ground black pepper and salt to taste

- 1 tsp. fresh lemon juice (or more if desired) to taste

- 3 tbsp. white wine vinegar

- 1/3 cup extra-virgin olive oil

Directions:

1. Get a bowl and whisk the pepper, salt, lemon juice, vinegar, and olive oil together until the dressing becomes smooth.

2. Next, get a large bowl and mix the garlic, parsley, red onion, and cauliflower. Then drizzle the dressing on top of the cauliflower mixture, toss together to have a coat. Fold the tomatoes inside the salad. Finally, place the salad inside the refrigerator and allow it to chill for at least 3 hours before you serve.

Nutrition:

- Calories: 157.7

- Protein: 3.2 g

- Carbs: 9.8 g

- Fats: 12.7 g

- Sodium: 46.9 mg

- Cholesterol: 0 mg

- Sugars: 3.7 g

24. Turkey Burger

Preparation Time: 15 minutes

Cooking Time: 10 minutes, **Additional Time:** 1 Hour 5 minutes

Servings: 4

Ingredients:

- 2 tbsp. chopped fresh cilantro

- 2 tbsp. plain yogurt

- 1 tbsp. lemon juice

- 1 ½ tsp. garam masala

- 1 ½ tsp. salt

- 1 ½ tsp. finely grated fresh ginger

- 2 garlic cloves, should be crushed and minced

- 1 tsp. Chile paste

- 1 ½ tbsp. ground almonds

- 1 ½ tbsp. plain bread crumbs

- 1 ½ lb. ground turkey

Directions:

1. Combine the cilantro, yogurt, lemon juice, garam masala, salt, ginger, garlic, chili paste, almonds, breadcrumbs, and ground turkey; mix very well with your clean hands or spatula.

2. Use the ground turkey mixture to form a ball shape, divide it into 4 even pieces, and then put in the refrigerator for an hour. Form patties with each of the pieces using your damp hands.

3. Get your grill preheated over medium heat and leave the turkey burger patties in the refrigerator until the grill becomes hot. Next is to grill the burgers until you observe that the patties are cooked halfway, and turn to the other side; you should grill each of its sides for about 5 minutes. The burger is said to be done when a crack appears on the surface, and its juice starts getting to the top.

Nutrition:

- Calories: 301.2
- Sodium: 1025.6 mg
- Protein: 34.4 g
- Cholesterol: 135.6 mg
- Carbs: 5 g
- Sugars: 1.2 g
- Fats: 16.3 g

25. Vegetable Tofu Soup with Coconut Milk and Lemongrass

Preparation Time: 40 minutes

Cooking Time: 33 minutes

Servings: 6

Ingredients:

- 1 (12 oz.) package medium-firm tofu, to be cubed and patted dry

- Salt to taste

- 2 tbsp. white sugar

- ¼ cup minced lemongrass

- ½ cup red lentils

- 2 ribs of celery, should be chopped

- 2 large carrots, should be cut into chunks

- 1 large yam, should be cut into chunks

- 1 (14 oz.) can of coconut milk

- 3 cups vegetable stock

- 2 tbsp. curry powder

- 1 tbsp. finely chopped ginger

- 1 tbsp. finely chopped garlic

- 1 large onion, to be chopped

- 5 tbsp. vegetable oil

Directions:

1. Get a large pot and pour 2 tbsp. oil, then place over medium heat, add onion, cook, and continuously stir it until it becomes brown in about 7 minutes. Stir in ginger and garlic and cook till it becomes fragrant in about 2 minutes. Add curry powder, cook, and continue to stir till it becomes fragrant in about 1 minute.

2. Pour coconut milk and vegetable stock inside the pot. Add sugar, lemongrass, lentils, celery, carrots, and yam. Raise the heat to medium-high and allow it to boil. Once it boils, reduce the heat a little bit and let it simmer until vegetables become soft in about 10–15 minutes and season with salt.

3. Get a large non-stick skillet and add the remaining 3 tbsp. of oil; place over medium heat. Place tofu in a single row

and let it cook until it becomes slightly brown in about 4 minutes for each side. Then, stir tofu inside the already prepared soup from step 2 above.

Nutrition:

- Calories: 475.1

- Protein: 12.4 g

- Carbs: 46 g

- Fats: 29.1 g

- Sodium: 218.9 mg

- Cholesterol: 0 mg

- Sugars: 7.8 g

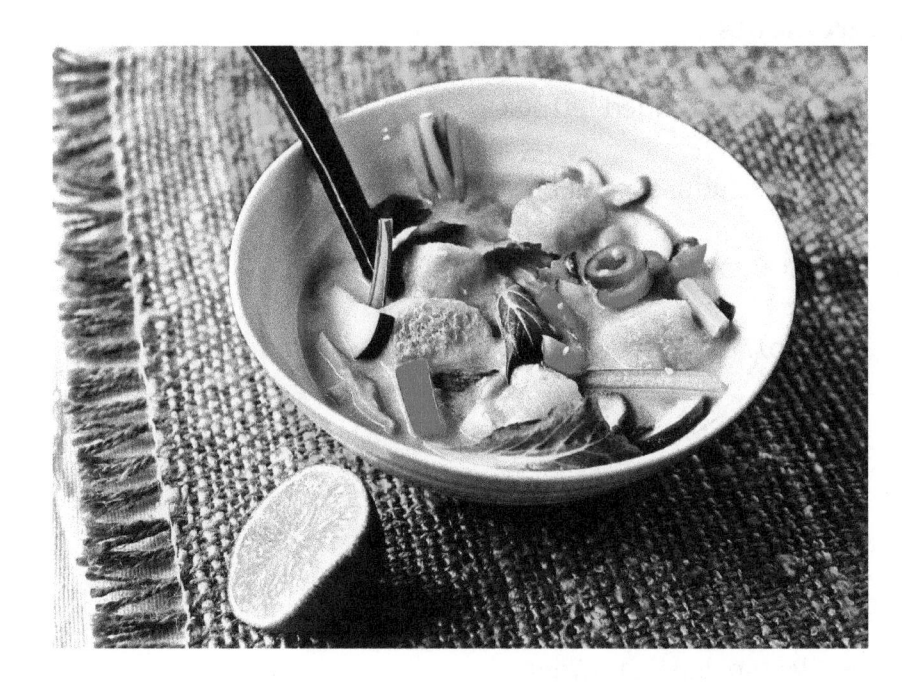

26. Black Bean Tacos

Preparation Time: 15 minutes

Cooking Time: 10 minutes

Servings: 4

Ingredients:

- 1 cup shredded lettuce

- 1 avocado, should be sliced

- 1 tomato, should be diced

- 2 oz. of shredded Mexican cheese, blend

- 6 units of taco shells

- ½ tsp. ground cumin

- ½ tsp. chili powder

- ½ tsp. garlic powder

- 1 (7 oz.) can "green salsa"

- 1 (15 oz.) can black beans, should be rinsed and drained

- 1 small onion, should be chopped

- 1 tbsp. olive oil

Directions:

1. Get a saucepan and pour in the olive oil, which should be heated over medium-low heat. Then, cook onion in the hot oil until it becomes tender in about 5 minutes. Stir the cumin, chili powder, garlic powder, green salsa and black beans with the onion. Lower the heat to low and cook the mixture till it becomes thicken in about 5–10 minutes.

2. Serve with shredded lettuce, avocado, tomato, Mexican cheese blend, and taco shells.

Nutrition:

- Calories: 402.1

- Protein: 13 g

- Carbs: 43.9 g

- Fats: 20.5 g

- Sodium: 778.1 mg

- Cholesterol: 13.5 mg

- Sugars: 4.4 g

27. Turmeric Chicken Stew

Preparation Time: 15 minutes

Cooking Time: 28 minutes

Servings: 6

Ingredients:

- ½ cup low-sodium chicken broth

- 2 tsp. ground turmeric

- 1 tbsp. minced fresh ginger root

- 2 garlic cloves, should be minced

- 1 small eggplant, should be cubed

- ½ red onion, should be chopped

- 2 units of sweet potatoes, should be cubed

- 2 breast half, the bone and skin should be removed, cubed

- 2 tbsp. olive oil

Directions:

1. Get a large skillet and pour the olive oil, then place it over medium-high heat. Add the chicken and let it cook till it is no longer pink at the center and becomes brown in about

5 minutes. Add onion and sweet potatoes, cook, and continue to stir until the onions become translucent in about 2–3 minutes. Add turmeric, ginger, garlic, and eggplant till it becomes fragrant (in a minute). Pour the broth over and let it simmer until the stew becomes thickened, and frequently stir for 20 minutes.

Nutrition:

- Calories: 183.1
- Protein: 9.9 g
- Carbs: 24.1 g
- Fats: 5.5 g
- Sodium: 70.8 mg
- Cholesterol: 20.3 mg
- Sugars: 5.7 g

28. Spicy Baked Tofu

Preparation Time: 10 minutes

Cooking Time: 30 minutes

Additional Time: 1 Hour 5 minutes

Servings: 4

Ingredients:

- 1 ½ tbsp. hoisin sauce

- 2 tbsp. minced fresh ginger root

- 2 tbsp. Asian chili sauce

- 2 tbsp. Japanese low-sodium soy sauce

- 1 (12 oz.) of package tofu

- 1 serving cooking spray

Directions:

1. Get a plate and line the tofu with some sheets of paper towel. Lay more paper towels on top of the tofu and put another plate on top of the stack to force out the tofu's water. Leave it for at least 5 minutes.

2. Cut the tofu into ½-inch strips, get a large sealable plastic bag, put the strips inside, and add hoisin sauce, ginger, chili sauce, and soy sauce. Squeeze the bag to get rid of the air trapped inside and seal. Then, let the tofu marinate in the refrigerator for about 1 hour.

3. Preheat your oven to 375°F (190°C). Get your baking sheet prepared with cooking spray.

4. You should now go ahead to remove the tofu from the marinade and shake very well to get rid of excessive moisture present, then gently place them on the baking sheet. You should throw away the remaining marinade.

5. Then bake in the already preheated oven for about 15 minutes and continue to bake till it becomes firm in about 15–20 minutes (it may take longer).

Nutrition:

- Calories: 87.9

- Protein: 7.4 g

- Carbs: 6.1 g

- Fats: 4.3 g

- Sodium: 686.2 mg

- Cholesterol: 0.2 mg

- Sugars: 2.2 g

29. Chicken with Veggies and Quinoa

Preparation Time: 30 minutes

Cooking Time: 25 minutes

Servings: 4

Ingredients:

- 1 tbsp. lime juice

- 8 leaves fresh basil leaves

- 4 oz. crumbled feta cheese

- 1 tomato, should be diced

- 1 zucchini, should be diced

- 2 tbsp. extra-virgin olive oil

- 2 breast half with the b1 and skin removed, should be cut into strips

- 1 small onion, should be chopped

- 2 units garlic scapes should be chopped.

- 2 tbsp. extra-virgin olive oil

- 2 cups chicken broth

- 1 cup rinsed quinoa

Directions:

1. Get a saucepan, add the chicken broth and quinoa, allow to boil, lower the heat to simmer level, and place a lid over the saucepan. Let it simmer until the white line is visible in the grain, the quinoa becomes fluffy, and the broth is absorbed in about 12 minutes.

2. Get a skillet and pour in 2 tbsp. of olive oil, heat it, cook and stir the onion and garlic scapes until the onion becomes translucent in 5 minutes. Add the chicken breast strips while stirring, and let it cook for about 5 minutes; the chicken should still be a little bit pink at the center from this point. At this point, remove the chicken meat and put it on 1 side.

3. Pour another 2 tbsp. of olive oil in the skillet and cook and stir the tomato and zucchini till the zucchini become tender in about 5–8 minutes. Put the chicken back inside the skillet and sprinkle with lime juice, basil leaves, and feta cheese. Cook for about 10 minutes when the chicken should be thoroughly cooked and hot. Serve with hot quinoa.

Nutrition:

- Calories: 445.3
- Protein: 23.3 g
- Carbs: 34.8 g
- Fats: 23.6 g

- Sodium: 361.4 mg
- Cholesterol: 58.8 mg
- Sugars: 3.6 g

30. Chicken Kabobs Mexicana

Preparation Time: 30 minutes

Cooking Time: 10 minutes

Additional Time: 1 Hour

Servings: 4

Ingredients:

- 10 units cherry tomatoes

- 1 red bell pepper, should be cut into 1-inch pieces

- 1 onion, should be cut into wedges and separated

- 1 small zucchini, should be cut into ½ - inch slices

- 2 breast half, with the b1 and skin removed

- Black pepper and salt to taste

- 1 lime, should be juiced

- 2 tbsp. chopped fresh cilantro

- 1 tsp. ground cumin

- 2 tbsp. olive oil

Directions:

1. Get a shallow dish and mix the lime juice, chopped cilantro, cumin, and olive oil inside. Then season with pepper and salt. Add the chicken, and make sure to mix it very well. Cover with a lid for not less than 1 hour.

2. Let your grill preheat over high heat.

3. Thread the tomatoes, red bell pepper, onion, zucchini, and chicken onto skewers.

4. Use oil to brush the grill and arrange the skewers on the hot grate. Let it cook for approximately 10 minutes till the chicken is thoroughly cooked. You should turn at intervals so that all sides of skewers are well cooked.

Nutrition:

- Calories: 165.8

- Protein: 15.2 g

- Carbs: 9.4 g

- Fats: 7.9 g

- Sodium: 49.4 mg

- Cholesterol: 34.2 mg

- Sugars: 3.2 g

106

Chapter 8: Fueling Recipes

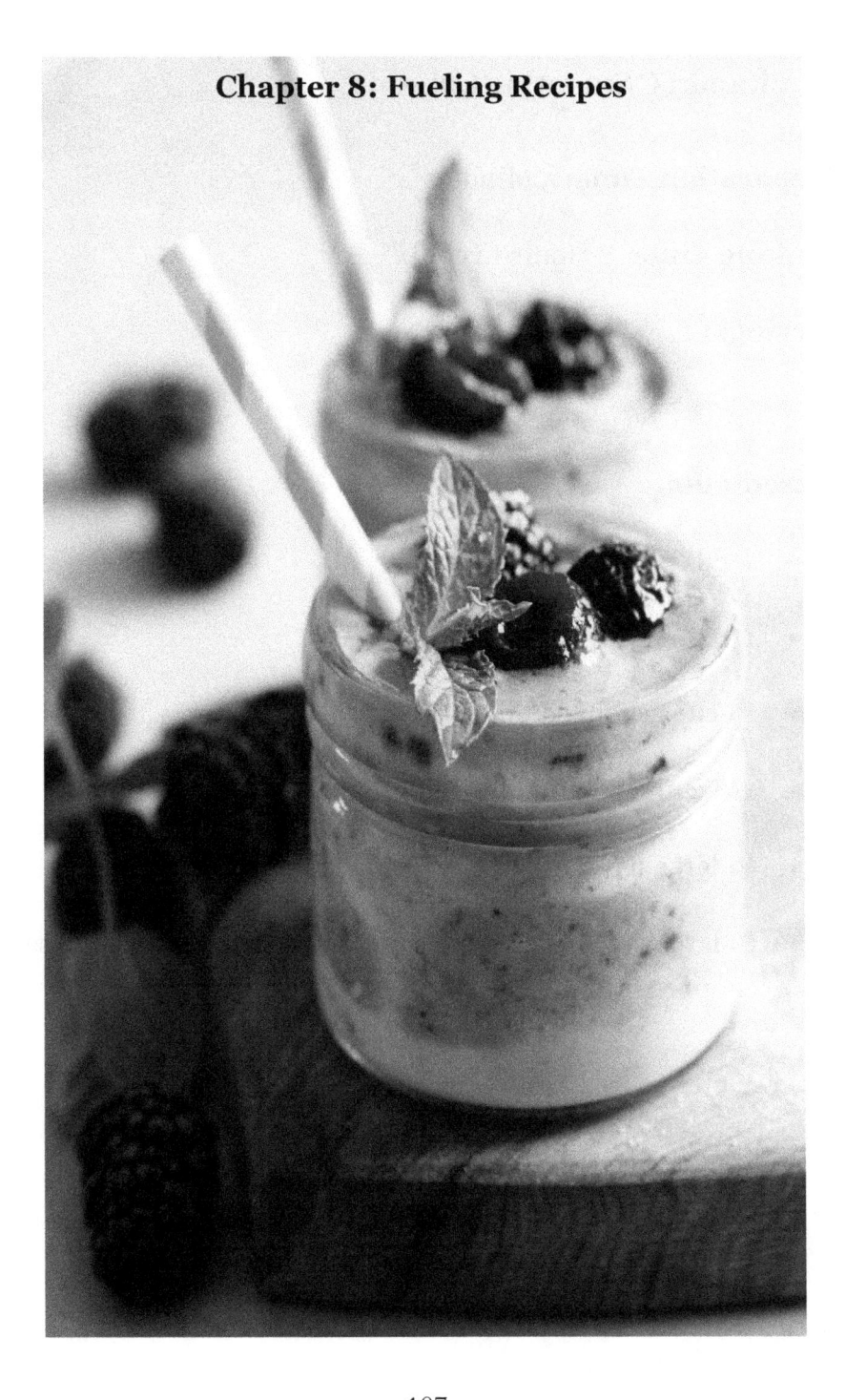

31. Vitamin C Smoothie Cubes

Preparation Time: 5 Minutes

Cooking Time: 8 Hours to chill

Servings: 1

Ingredients:

- 1/8 large papaya

- 1/8 mango

- ¼ cups chopped pineapple, fresh or frozen

- 1/8 cup raw cauliflower florets, fresh or frozen

- ¼ large navel oranges, peeled and halved

- ¼ large orange bell pepper stemmed, seeded, and coarsely chopped

Directions:

1. Halve the papaya and mango, remove the pits, and scoop their soft flesh into a high-speed blender.

2. Add the pineapple, cauliflower, oranges, and bell pepper. Blend until smooth.

3. Evenly divide the purée between 2 (16-compartment) ice cube trays and place them on a leveled surface in your freezer. Freeze for at least 8 hours.

4. The cubes can be left in the ice cube trays or transferred to a freezer bag. The frozen cubes are good for about 3 weeks in a standard freezer or up to 6 months in a chest freezer.

Nutrition:

- Calories: 96
- Carbs: 24 g
- Fats: <1 g
- Fiber: 4 g
- Protein: 2 g

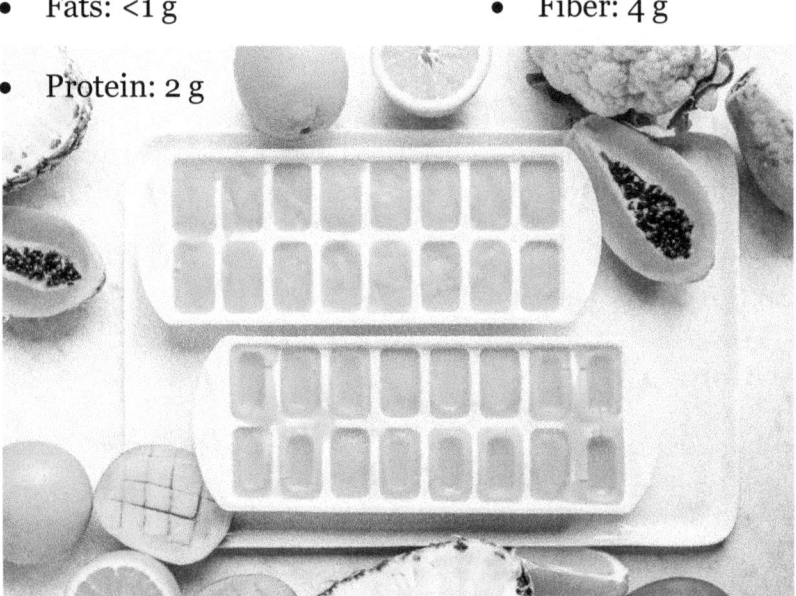

32. Overnight Chocolate Chia Pudding

Preparation Time: 2 Minutes

Cooking Time: Overnight to Chill

Servings: 1

Ingredients:

- 1/8 cup chia seeds

- ½ cup unsweetened nondairy milk

- 1 tbsp. raw cacao powder

- ½ tsp. vanilla extract

- ½ tsp. pure maple syrup

Directions:

1. Stir together the chia seeds, milk, cacao powder, vanilla, and maple syrup in a large bowl. Divide between 2 (½-pint) covered glass jars or containers. Refrigerate overnight.

2. Stir before serving.

Nutrition:

- Calories: 213

- Fats: 10 g

- Protein: 9 g

- Carbs: 20 g

- Fiber: 15 g

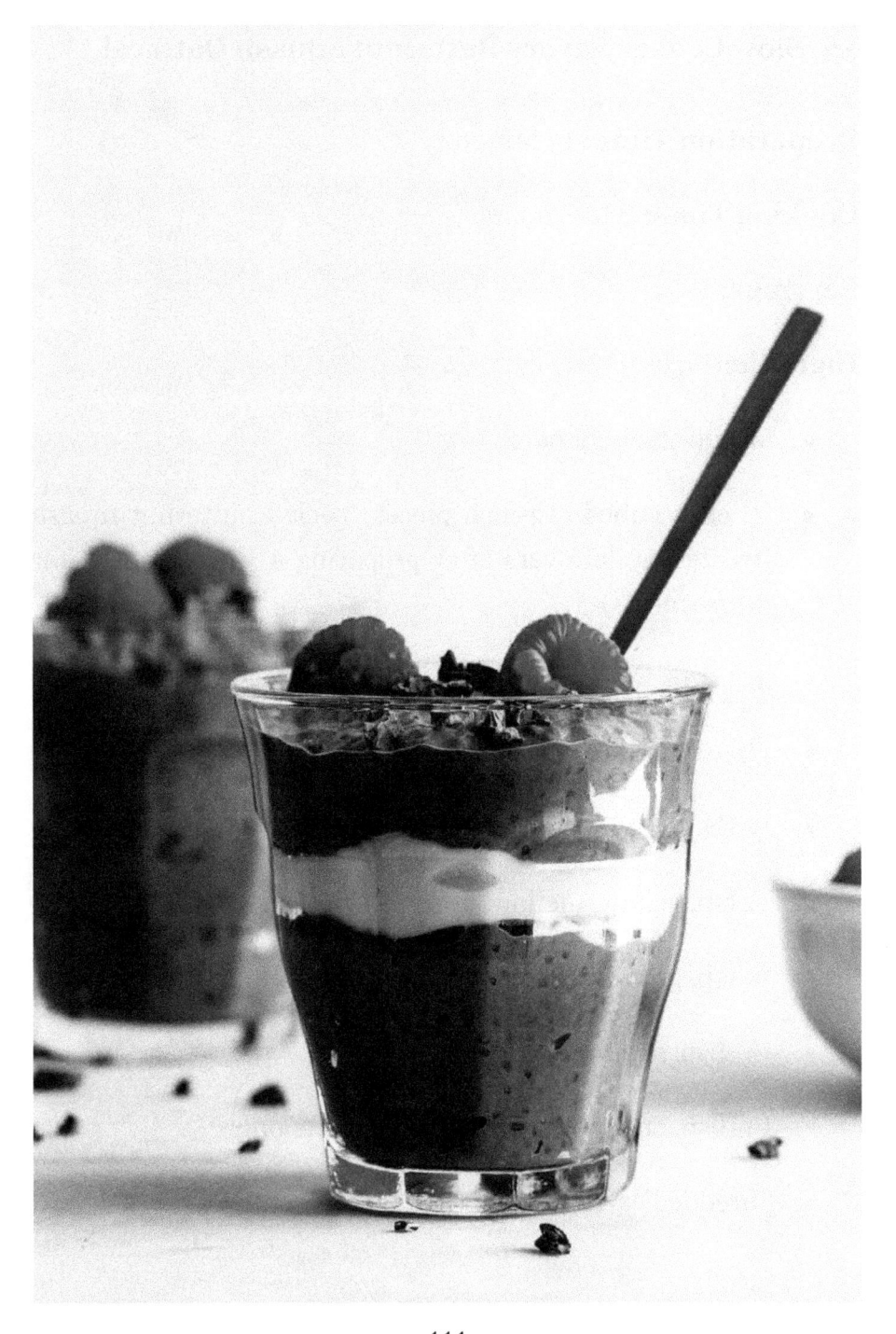

33. Slow Cooker Savory Butternut Squash Oatmeal

Preparation Time: 15 Minutes

Cooking Time: 6 to 8 hours

Servings: 1

Ingredients:

- ¼ cup steel-cut oats

- ½ cups cubed (½-inch pieces) peeled butternut squash (freeze any leftovers after preparing a whole squash for future meals)

- 3/4 cups water

- 1/16 cup unsweetened nondairy milk

- ¼ tbsp. chia seed

- ½ tsp. yellow, mellow, miso paste

- ¾ tsp. ground ginger

- ¼ tbsp. sesame seed, toasted

- ¼ tbsp. chopped scallion, green parts only

- Shredded carrot, for serving, optional

Directions:

1. In a slow cooker, combine the oats, butternut squash, and water.

2. Cover the slow cooker and cook on low for 6 to 8 hours, or until the squash is fork tender. Using a potato masher or heavy spoon, roughly mash the cooked butternut squash. Stir to combine with the oats.

3. Whisk together the milk, chia seeds, miso paste, and ginger to combine in a large bowl. Stir the mixture into the oats.

4. Top your oatmeal bowl with sesame seeds and scallion for more plant-based fiber, top with shredded carrot (if using).

Nutrition:

- Calories: 230

- Fats: 5 g

- Protein: 7 g

- Carbs: 40 g

- Fiber: 9 g

34. Carrot Cake Oatmeal

Preparation Time: 10 Minutes

Cooking Time: 15 Minutes

Servings: 1

Ingredients:

- 1/8 cup pecans

- ½ cup finely shredded carrot

- ¼ cup old-fashi1d oats

- 5/8 cups unsweetened nondairy milk

- ½ tbsp. pure maple syrup

- ½ tsp. ground cinnamon

- ½ tsp. ground ginger

- 1/8 tsp. ground nutmeg

- 1 tbsp. chia seed

Directions:

1. Over medium-high heat, in a skillet, toast the pecans for 3 to 4 minutes, often stirring, until browned and fragrant

(watch closely, as they can burn quickly). Pour the pecans onto a cutting board and coarsely chop them. Set aside.

2. In an 8-quart pot over medium-high heat, combine the carrot, oats, milk, maple syrup, cinnamon, ginger, and nutmeg. When it is already boiling, reduce the heat to medium-low. Cook, uncovered, for 10 minutes, stirring occasionally.

3. Stir in the chopped pecans and chia seeds. Serve immediately.

Nutrition:

- Calories: 307
- Carbs: 35 g
- Fats: 17 g
- Fiber: 11 g
- Protein: 7 g

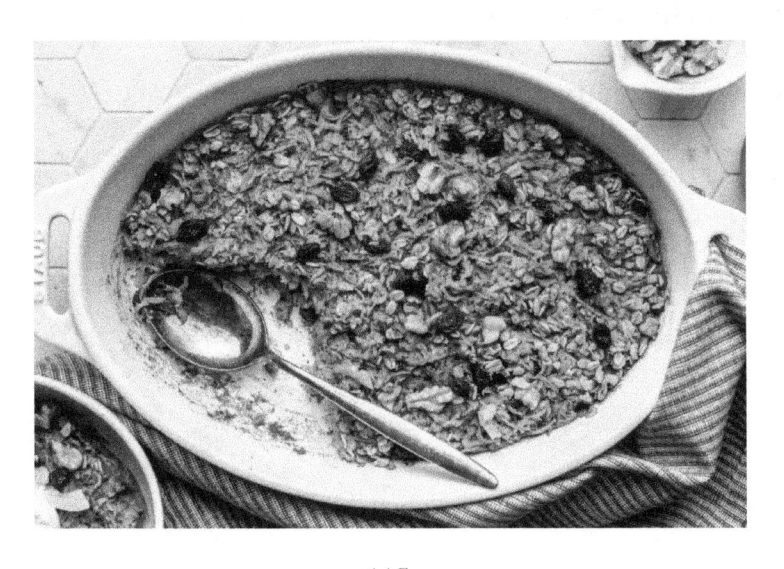

35. Spiced Sorghum and Berries

Preparation Time: 5 Minutes

Cooking Time: 1 hour

Servings: 1

Ingredients:

- ¼ cup whole-grain sorghum

- ¼ tsp. ground cinnamon

- ¼ tsp. Chinese 5-spice powder

- ¾ cups water

- ¼ cup unsweetened nondairy milk

- ¼ tsp. vanilla extract

- ½ tbsp. pure maple syrup

- ½ tbsp. chia seed

- 1/8 cup sliced almonds

- ½ cups fresh raspberries, divided

Directions:

1. Using a large pot over medium-high heat, stir together the sorghum, cinnamon, 5-spice powder, and water. Wait for the water to boil, cover the bank, and reduce the heat to medium-low. Cook for 1 hour, or until the sorghum is soft and chewy. If the sorghum grains are still hard, add another water cup and cook for 15 minutes more.

2. Using a glass measuring cup, whisk together the milk, vanilla, and maple syrup to blend. Add the mixture to the sorghum and the chia seeds, almonds, and 1 cup raspberries. Gently stir to combine.

3. When serving, top with the remaining 1 cup fresh raspberries.

Nutrition:

- Calories: 289

- Fats: 8 g

- Protein: 9 g

- Carbs: 52 g

- Fiber: 10 g

36. Raw-Cinnamon-Apple Nut Bowl

Preparation Time: 15 Minutes

Cooking Time: 1 Hour to Chill

Servings: 1

Ingredients:

- 1 green apple, halved, seeded, and cored

- 3/4 honey-crisp apples, halved, seeded, and cored

- ¼ tsp. freshly squeezed lemon juice

- 1 pitted Medrol dates

- 1/8 tsp. ground cinnamon

- Pinch ground nutmeg

- ½ tbsp. chia seeds, plus more for serving, optional

- ¼ tbsp. hemp seed

- 1/8 cup chopped walnuts

- Nut butter, for serving, optional

Directions:

1. Finely dice half the green apple and 1 Honey crisp apple. With the lemon juice, store it in an air-tight container while you work on the next steps.

2. Coarsely chop the remaining apples and the Medrol dates. Transfer to a food processor and add the cinnamon and nutmeg. Check several times if it combines, then process for 2 to 3 minutes to purée. Stir the purée into the reserved diced apples. Stir in the chia seeds (if using), hemp seeds, and walnuts. Chill for at least 1 hour.

3. Serve as is or top with additional chia seeds and nut butter (if using).

4. Enjoy!

Nutrition:

- Calories: 274

- Fats: 8 g

- Protein: 4 g

- Carbs: 52 g

- Fiber: 9 g

37. Peanut Butter and Cacao Breakfast Quinoa

Preparation Time: 5 Minutes

Cooking Time: 10 Minutes

Servings: 1

Ingredients:

- 1/3 cup quinoa flakes

- ½ cup unsweetened nondairy milk,

- ½ cup water

- 1/8 cup raw cacao powder

- 1 tbsp. natural creamy peanut butter

- 1/8 tsp. ground cinnamon

- 1 banana, mashed

- Fresh berries of choice, for serving

- Chopped nuts of choice, for serving

Directions:

1. Using an 8-quart pot over medium-high heat, stir together the quinoa flakes, milk, water, cacao powder, peanut butter, and cinnamon. Cook and stir until the mixture

begins to simmer. Turn the heat to medium-low and cook for 3 to 5 minutes, stirring frequently.

2. Stir in the bananas and cook until hot.

3. Serve topped with fresh berries, nuts, and a splash of milk.

Nutrition:

- Calories: 471
- Carbs: 69 g
- Fats: 16 g
- Fiber: 16 g
- Protein: 18 g

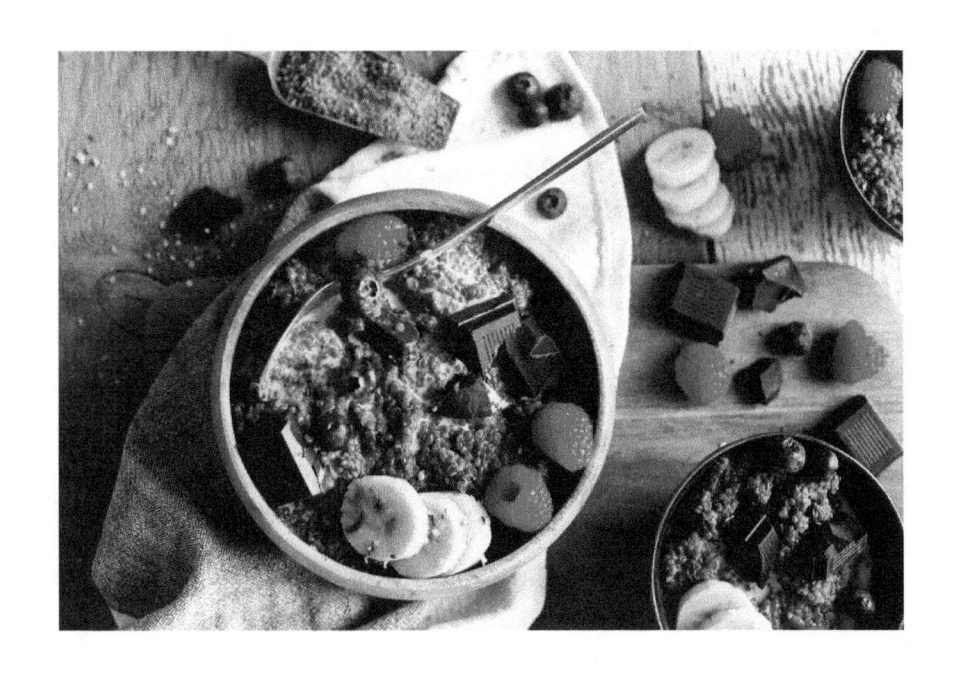

38. Vanilla Buckwheat Porridge

Preparation Time: 5 Minutes

Cooking Time: 25 Minutes

Servings: 1

Ingredients:

- 1 cup water

- ¼ cup raw buckwheat grout

- ¼ tsp. ground cinnamon

- ¼ banana, sliced

- 1/16 cup golden raisins

- 1/16 cup dried currant

- 1/16 cup sunflower seed

- ½ tbsp. chia seed

- ¼ tbsp. hemp seed

- ¼ tbsp. sesame seed, toasted

- 1/8 cup unsweetened nondairy milk

- ¼ tbsp. pure maple syrup

- ¼ tsp. vanilla extract

Directions:

1. Boil the water in a pot. Stir in the buckwheat, cinnamon, and banana. Cook the mixture. Mix it and wait for it to boil, then reduce the heat to medium-low. Cover the pot and

cook for 15 minutes, or until the buckwheat is tender. Remove from the heat.

2. Stir in the raisins, currants, sunflower seeds, chia seeds, hemp seeds, sesame seeds, milk, maple syrup, and vanilla. Cover the pot. Wait for 10 minutes before serving.

3. Serve as is or top as desired.

Nutrition:

- Calories: 353
- Carbs: 61 g
- Fats: 11 g
- Fiber: 10 g
- Protein: 10 g

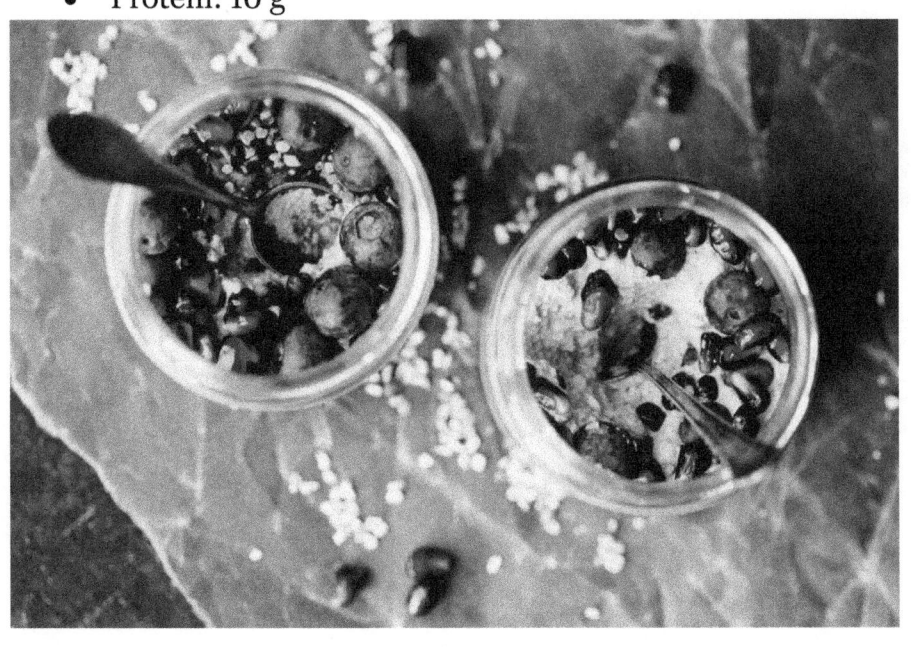

39. Polenta with Seared Pears

Preparation Time: 10 Minutes

Cooking Time: 50 Minutes

Servings: 1

Ingredients:

- 1 cup water, divided, plus more as needed

- ½ cup coarse cornmeal

- 1 tbsp. pure maple syrup

- ¼ tbsp. molasses

- ¼ tsp. ground cinnamon

- ½ ripe pear, cored and diced

- ¼ cup fresh cranberries

- ¼ tsp. chopped fresh rosemary leaves

Directions:

1. In a pan, bring 5 cups of water to a simmer.

2. While whisking continuously to avoid clumping, slowly pour in the cornmeal. Cook, often stirring with a heavy

spoon, for 30 minutes. The polenta should be thick and creamy.

3. While the polenta cooks, in a saucepan over medium heat, stir together the maple syrup, molasses, the remaining ¼ cup water, and the cinnamon until combined. Bring it to a simmer. Add the pears and cranberries. Cook for 10 minutes, occasionally stirring until the pears are tender and start to brown. Remove from the heat. Stir in the rosemary and let the mixture sit for 5 minutes. If it is too thick, add another ¼ cup water and return to the heat.

4. Top with the cranberry-pear mixture.

Nutrition:

- Calories: 282

- Fats: 2 g

- Protein: 4 g

- Carbs: 65 g

- Fiber: 12 g

40. Best Whole Wheat Pancakes

Preparation Time: 10 Minutes

Cooking Time: 20 Minutes

Servings: 1

Ingredients:

- ¾ tbsp. ground flaxseed

- 2 tbsp. warm water

- ½ cups whole wheat pastry flour

- 1/8 cup rye flour

- ½ tbsp. double-acting baking powder

- ¼ tsp. ground cinnamon

- 1/8 tsp. ground ginger

- 1 cup unsweetened nondairy milk

- ¾ tbsp. pure maple syrup

- ¼ tsp. vanilla extract

Directions:

1. Mix the warm water and flaxseed in a large bowl. Set aside for at least 5 minutes.

2. Whisk together the pastry, rye flours, baking powder, cinnamon, and ginger.

3. Whisk together the milk, maple syrup, and vanilla in a large bowl. Make use of a spatula, fold the wet ingredients into the dry ingredients. Fold in the soaked flaxseed until fully incorporated.

4. Heat a large skillet or nonstick griddle over medium-high heat. Working in batches, 3 to 4 pancakes at a time, add ¼-cup portions of batter to the hot skillet. Until golden brown, cook for 3 to 4 minutes each side or no liquid batter is visible.

Nutrition:

- Calories: 301

- Fats: 4 g

- Protein: 10 g

- Carbs: 57 g

- Fiber: 10 g

41. Spiced Pumpkin Muffins

Preparation Time: 15 Minutes

Cooking Time: 20 Minutes

Servings: 1

Ingredients:

- 1/6 tbsp. ground flaxseed

- 4 ½ cup water

- 1/8 cup whole wheat flour

- 1/6 tsp. baking powder

- 5/6 tsp. ground cinnamon

- 1/12 tsp. baking soda

- 1/12 tsp. ground ginger

- 1/16 tsp. ground nutmeg

- 1/32 tsp. ground cloves

- 1/6 cup pumpkin purée

- 1/12 cup pure maple syrup

- 4 ½ cup unsweetened applesauce

- 4 ½ cup unsweetened nondairy milk

- ½ tsp. vanilla extract

Directions:

1. Preheat the oven to 350°F (177°C). Line a 12-cup metal muffin pan with parchment paper liners or use a silicone muffin pan.

2. First, mix the flaxseeds and water in a large bowl, then keep it aside.

3. In a medium bowl, stir together the flour, baking powder, cinnamon, baking soda, ginger, nutmeg, and cloves.

4. In a medium bowl, stir up the maple syrup, pumpkin purée, applesauce, milk, and vanilla. Crease the wet ingredients into the dry ingredients (make use of a spatula).

5. Fold the soaked flaxseed into the batter until evenly combined, but do not over mix the batter, or your muffins will become dense. Spoon about ¼ cup batter per muffin into your prepared muffin pan.

6. Bake for 18 to 20 minutes, or until a toothpick inserted into the center of a muffin comes out clean. Remove the muffins from the pan.

7. Transfer to a wire rack for cooling.

8. Store in an air-tight container that is at room temperature.

Nutrition:

- Calories: 115

- Fats: 1 g

- Protein: 3 g

- Carbs: 25 g

- Fiber: 3 g

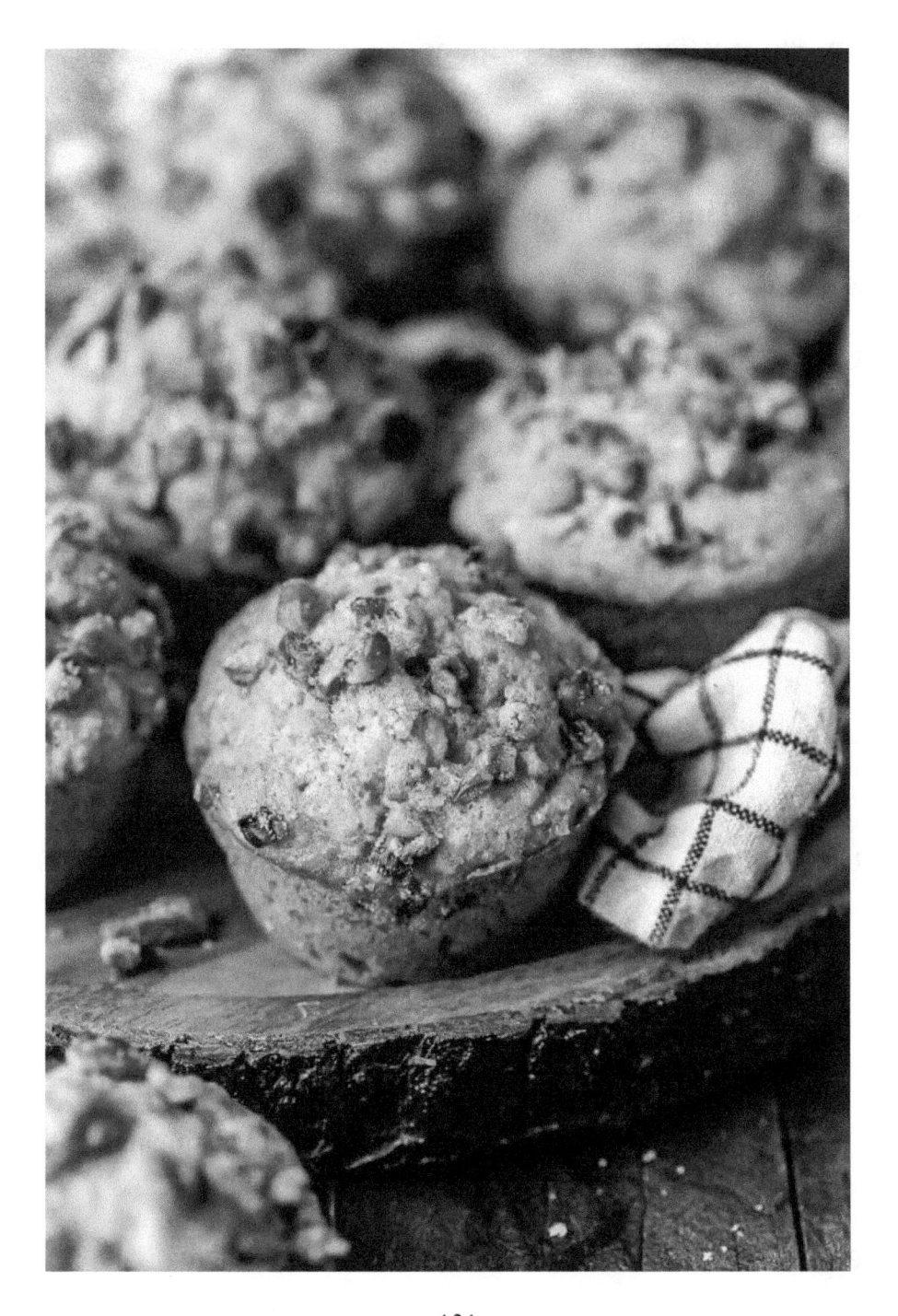

42. Skinny Peppermint Mocha

Preparation Time: 5 minutes

Cooking Time: 0 minutes

Servings: 1

Ingredients:

- 1 Pinch cinnamon

- 2 tbsp. pressurized whipped topping

- ¼ tsp. peppermint extract

- ¼ cup unsweetened cashew milk or vanilla almond, should be warmed

- 6 oz. freshly brewed coffee

- 1 Package Essential Velvety Hot Chocolate

Directions:

1. Get a coffee cup or mug to combine the cashew milk or vanilla almond, brewed coffee, and Velvety Hot Chocolate and stir everything together until the Velvety Hot Chocolate dissolves.

2. Top it with the whipped topping and spread cinnamon at the top.

Per Servings: 1 ½ Condiment, and 1 Fueling.

43. Egg & Cheese Bagel Sandwich

Preparation Time: 10 minutes

Cooking Time: 5 minutes

Servings: 1

Ingredients:

- 1 slice reduced-fat cheddar cheese

- 1 egg

- 1 tsp. everything bagel seasoning

- Cooking spray

- 3 tbsp. cold water

- 1 Package Optavia Select Buttermilk Cheddar Herb Biscuit

Directions:

1. Preheat your oven to 350°F (177°C).

2. Combine water and biscuits and mix very well before diving the mixture equally in 2 slots of the donut pan. Drizzle the top with seasoning and bake for 12–15 minutes when the edges should have become golden brown.

3. Get a lightly greased skillet to cook the egg.

4. Top 1 of the "bagel" piece with the egg and cheese before topping it with the other "bagel" piece.

Per Servings: 3 Condiments, 1 Fueling, and ½ Lean.

44. Boo-Nila Shake

Preparation Time: 5 minutes

Cooking Time: 0 minutes

Servings: 1

Ingredients:

- 2 tbsp. pressurized whipped topping

- ½ cup ice

- 8 oz. unsweetened cashew milk or vanilla almond

- 1 package Essential Creamy Vanilla Shake

Directions:

1. Get a blender to combine the ice, cashew milk or vanilla almond, and Creamy Vanilla Shake and blend everything together till they become smooth.

2. You can use a black permanent marker to decorate a plastic/glass cup or mason jar and have a ghost face on it (this is optional). Then, top with the whipped topping before serving.

Per Servings: 2 Condiments and 1 Fueling.

45. Cheesy Spinach Smashed Potatoes

Preparation Time: 10 minutes

Cooking Time: 0 minutes

Servings: 1

Ingredients:

- 1 tbsp. grated Parmesan cheese

- ½ cup reduced-Fat shredded mozzarella cheese

- 1 tsp. water

- 1 cup baby Spinach

- 1 package Essential Roasted Garlic Creamy Smashed Potatoes

Directions:

1. Check the package conditions for guidelines on how you will preheat the Roasted Garlic Creamy Smashed Potatoes. Put the spinach and water inside the microwave and steam for a minute or until it becomes wilted.

2. Combine the Parmesan, mozzarella, spinach, and Roasted Garlic Creamy Smashed Potatoes.

Per Servings: 1 Condiment, 1 Fueling, ½ Lean, 1 Green, and 1 Healthy Fat.

46. Tropical Smoothie Bowl

Preparation Time: 5 minutes

Cooking Time: 0 minutes

Servings: 1

Ingredients:

- ½ tsp. lime zest

- ½ tbsp. chia seeds

- 1 tbsp. shredded, unsweetened coconut

- ½ oz. cashews or macadamias, should be chopped

- ½ cup ice

- ½ cup unsweetened, original coconut milk

- 1 package Essential Tropical Fruit Smoothie

Directions:

1. Get a blender and add ice, milk, and the Tropical Fruit Smoothie and then blend until they become smooth.

2. Pour the formed smoothie inside a small bowl.

3. Finally, top with the rest of the ingredients and serve.

Per Servings: 2 ½ Condiments, 1 Fueling, and 2 Healthy Fats.

47. Hamburger Mac

Preparation Time: 10 minutes

Cooking Time: 0 minutes

Servings: 1

Ingredients:

- ¼ tsp. onion powder

- ¼ tsp. garlic powder

- ¼ tsp. chili powder

- 3 oz. cooked 95–97% lean ground beef

- ½ tbsp. tomato paste

- 1 package Cheesy Buttermilk Mac

Directions:

1. Check the package instruction of the Cheesy Buttermilk Mac for guidelines on how to prepare it.

2. With the Mac still hot, add tomato paste and stir until they are smooth. Then stir in seasonings with beef.

Per Servings: 3 Condiments, 1 Fueling, and ½ Lean.

48. Shrimp Cobb Salad

Preparation Time: 10 minutes

Cooking Time: 0 minutes

Servings: 1

Ingredients:

- 1 tbsp. light Ranch dressing

- 1/8 avocado, should be diced

- 1 slice turkey bacon, should be chopped

- 1 hard-boiled egg, should be sliced

- ½ cup grape or cherry tomatoes, should be halved

- 4 oz. cooked and peeled shrimp

- 2 cups romaine lettuce

- 1 package Puffed Ranch Snacks

Directions:

1. Get a medium-size bowl and combine the avocado, turkey bacon, egg, tomatoes, shrimp, and lettuce.

2. Top the salad with Puffed Ranch Snacks and dressing, serve immediately.

Per Servings: 1 Healthy Fat: 3 Green, 1 Leaner, and 1 Optional Snack.

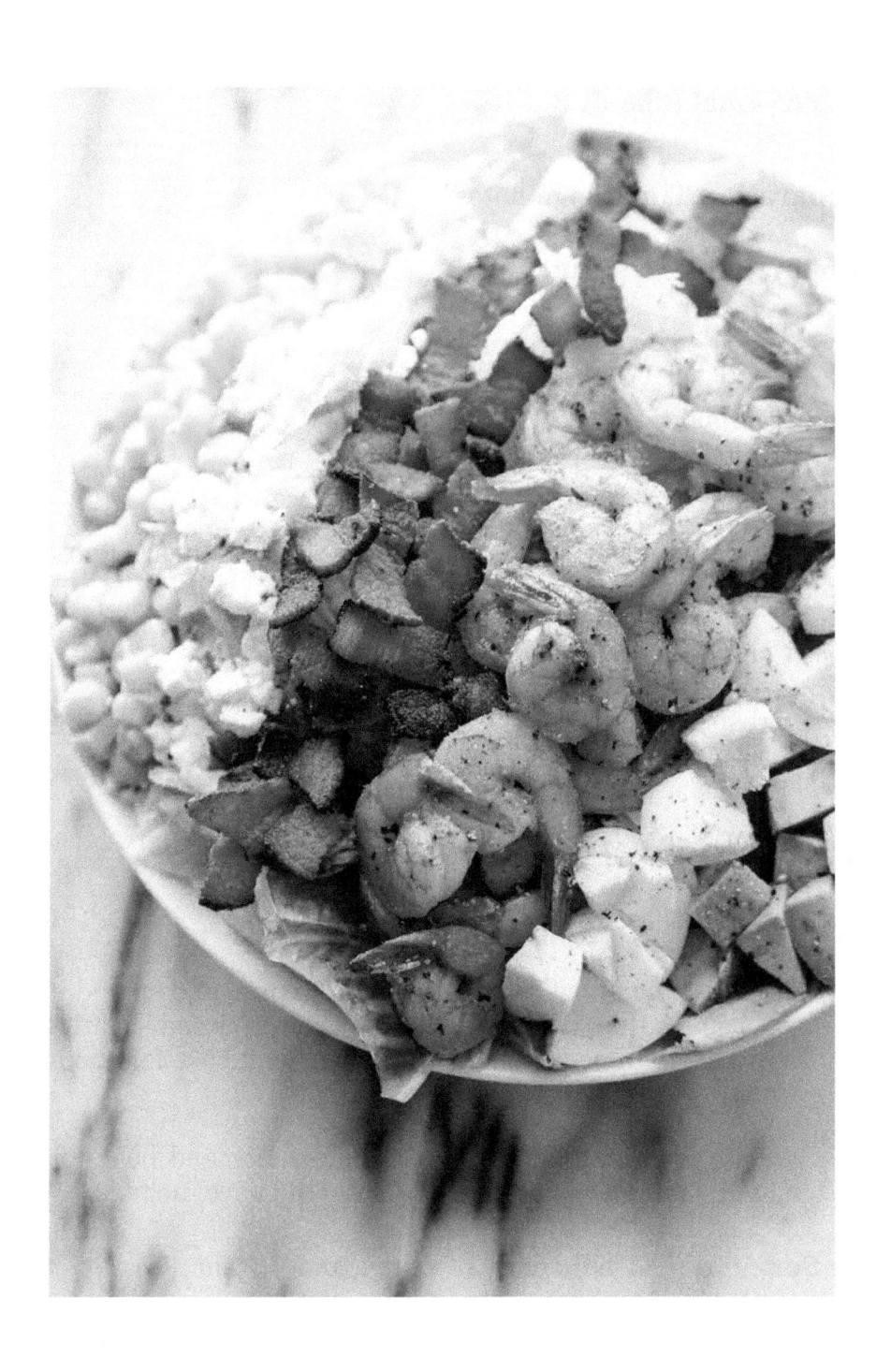

49. Personal Biscuit Pizza

Preparation Time: 15 minutes

Cooking Time: 0 minutes

Servings: 1

Ingredients:

- ¼ cup reduced-fat shredded cheese

- 2 tbsp. no-sugar-added tomato sauce, an example is Rao's Homemade

- Cooking spray

- 2 tbsp. cold water

- 1 package Select Buttermilk Cheddar Herb Biscuit

Directions:

1. Preheat your oven to 350°F.

2. Mix the biscuit with water to get a mixture, and spread it on a small, thin, circular crust shape in the already lightly-greased, foil-lined baking sheet. Then, let it bake for about 10 minutes.

3. Finally, top with cheese and tomato sauce and bake for about 5 minutes when the cheese should have melted.

Per Servings: 2 Condiments, 1 Fueling, and ¼ Lean.

50. 2-Ingredient Peanut Butter Energy Bites

Preparation Time: 5 minutes

Cooking Time: 0 minutes

Servings: 1

Ingredients:

- 1 tbsp. water

- 2 tbsp. powdered peanut butter

- 1 Essential Cream Double Peanut Butter Crisp Bar

Directions:

1. Get a small bowl to mix the powdered peanut butter with water and have a smooth paste.

2. Put the Creamy Double Peanut Butter Crisp Bar inside a microwave-safe plate and let it cook for about 15 seconds or till it becomes soft.

3. Next is to combine the peanut butter with warm pieces of the bar to get a dough.

4. Use your fingers or cookie scoop to form 4 bite-sized balls. You should keep them in the refrigerator until you are ready to serve.

Per Servings: 1 Fueling, and 1 Optional Snack.

142

Conclusion

The Low Carb Lean and Green Diet has been subjected to various studies to prove its efficacy in weight loss. Different studies were published in various journals indicating that those who follow this program can see significant changes in as little as 8 weeks and that people can achieve their long-term health goals with the Carb Lean and Green Diet.

While the Initial 5&1 Ideal Weight Plan is quite restrictive, maintenance phases of the 3&3 Plan allow for a greater variety of less processed foods and snacks, which can facilitate weight loss.

Under this diet regimen, dieters are required to follow a weight plan that includes 5 fuelings a day and 1 Lean and Green meal daily. However, there are also other regimens of the Low Carb Lean and Green Diet if the 5 fuelings a day is too much for you.

The diet is a set of 3 programs, 2 of which focus on weight loss and 1 that is best for weight maintenance if you are not trying to lose weight. The plans are high in protein and low in carbohydrates and calories to stimulate weight loss

Since the plan requires the intake of carbohydrates, protein, and fat, it is also a relatively balanced plan when it comes to food groups.

When it comes to weight loss, experts say that while Low Carb Lean and Green can help because it is essentially less caloric, it is unlikely to permanently improve your eating habits. You are more likely to gain weight after stopping the diet.

Also, diet experts warn that this pattern may not contain enough calories to meet your body's needs. "In terms of overall health and nutrition, as well as convenience, this diet isn't at the top of my list of best approaches."—London says.

If you are interested in trying this, consider working with an experienced, registered dietitian who can help you stay properly fed as you strive to achieve your desired weight.

For the most desirable 5&1 Weight Plan, eat 5 foods per day, plus a low carb lean meal and a low carb elective snack.

Although the initial 5&1 Plan is reasonably restrictive, Protection segments of the 3&3 Plan allow for a greater variety of less processed foods and snacks, which can also make weight loss easier and more persistent for a long period.

The bottom line is that the Carb Lean and Green weight loss plan promotes weight loss via low-calorie and low carb homemade food; at the same time, as this system promotes quick-time period weight and fat loss, similarly research is wanted to assess whether it encourages the everlasting way of life adjustments needed for long-lasting achievements.

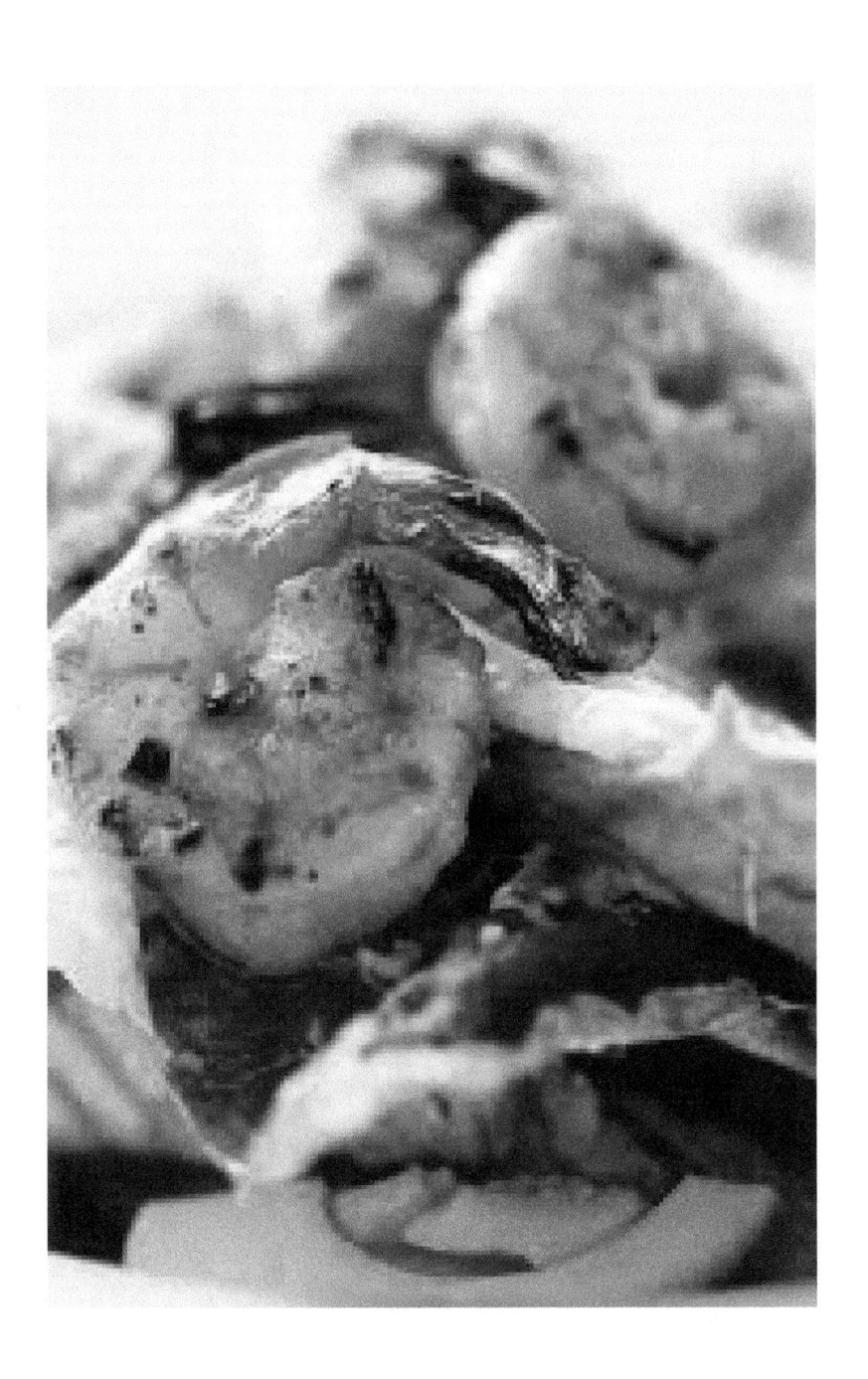